Never Grow Old!

The innovative, easy to follow functional aging fitness program that increases strength, improves balance and decreases pain

By :

Dan Ritchie, PhD

&

Cody Sipe, PhD

ISBN-13: **978-1497584754**

ISBN-10: **1497584752**

To contact our company directly:

Functional Fitness Solution
257 Sagamore Pkwy W, Ste B
West Lafayette, IN 47906

Visit us online for fitness programs
www.functionalfitnesssolution.com

For Fitness Professionals

www.functionalaginginstitute.com

Acknowledgements

We want to thank our wives and family for their support, commitment, and love since we started this journey. They have seen us through the stresses of starting and building a business (while finishing up PhD's with multiple children at home).

We are very thankful to have had great mentors, teachers, colleagues, and friends along the way. Their expertise, professionalism, and guidance has been more valuable then they will ever know. To Roseann Lyle, PhD, who saw us both through to completion of our degrees, how you kept two dreamers like us on task to complete PhDs is quite remarkable!

None of this would have been possible without all of the great clients (who have become friends) that we have had the opportunity to train and, at times, experiment on.

Special thanks go to the exercise models who volunteered their time and effort to help make this book.

Lastly, but most importantly, we thank God who has made all of this possible.

Table of Contents

Core Principles
Introduction

Chapters	Page
1. Dysfunctional Exercise	3
2. The Never Grow Old Fitness Formula	15
3. The Never Grow Old Program	29
4. Functional Fitness Workouts	45
5. No More Low and Slow (and boring) Cardio	133
6. Holding Your Own	143
7. Conclusion	153

Our Core Principles

We Believe:

- Aging is mandatory…but growing old is optional
- Improving functional fitness is critical to living a long, healthy and enjoyable life
- Traditional resistance training does NOT maximize function
- Exercise is a powerful stimulus with numerous benefits
- It is NEVER too late to begin a fitness program and reap its benefits
- If you move better you will feel better. If you feel better you will move more. If you move more you will look better.
- Fitness is one of the best investments of time, money and effort that a mature adult can make and it will yield huge benefits
- All exercise programs are NOT created equal!

Our Mission is to help people achieve the best possible health and quality of life through innovative and evidence-based functional fitness programs that are safe, effective, enjoyable and purposeful.

Introduction

In my office is a framed poster-size black and white photograph of an older gentleman with his shirt off holding a set of dumbbells. He has receding gray hair and a white moustache and goatee. His sweats are the gray "old school" sweats people used to wear 30 years ago. You know the kind, with the drawstring tied in the front hanging out where you can see it. He has a very wrinkled face and clear, intelligent eyes. But what is striking about the picture is the juxtaposition of the gentleman's older looking face with his body. His torso is muscular and lean. His chest and shoulders are prominent and developed. His abdominal muscles are clearly defined. A vein can be readily traced down both arms like you see in many athletes. He doesn't look like a body builder or someone on steroids but simply fit and strong. It's almost as if the head of an older man was photo shopped onto the body of someone much younger. Yet, this is an actual photograph of a 67 year old psychiatrist.*

I speak to older audiences about the benefits of exercise and being fit I often show them this picture with the head cropped off so you cannot see above his neck. Most people in the audience assume that this is the body of a 25 or 30 year old and are rather dismissive of the picture thinking "that could never be me". When I show the whole picture, so they can see the apparent age of this man, people are surprised. It is difficult for them to believe that a man that old could look so good (lean and fit that is). But what I love the most about this picture is the subtitle which reads "Growing Old Is Not For Sissies"*.

I love that phrase and I love that attitude. In fact, it really encompasses what this book is all about. You have a lot of influence over how you age. You can choose to perpetuate the stereotype that older people are sick, weak and tired by sitting back and doing nothing to prepare for the coming years (the path of "sissies") or you can choose to chart your own path. One that isn't for "sissies". You're ready and willing to make the final third of your life's journey even more fulfilling, more vibrant, more purposeful, more meaningful, more pleasurable and more engaged than the first two-thirds. You've chosen to tell the world "I WILL NEVER GROW OLD!"

And this is where we come in. Over the years, Dan and I have helped thousands of middle-aged and older adults improve the quality of their life through transformational exercise programs that maximize physical function. Our goal is always to help clients look better, feel better and, most importantly, move better. It is the move better part that is at the core of what we do. If people can move better then they start to feel better. And if they feel better they move more. And, if they move more, then eventually they start to look better as well (by losing body fat and building muscle).

Now we want to help you experience these amazing results. We hope that by following the exercise principles and techniques contained in this book your life will be enriched.

    - Cody Sipe, PhD

* This picture was originally included in a book of the same name by photographer Etta Clark. The book is full of pictures of amazing active older adults like 83 year old surfer Woody Brown and 76 year old weightlifter Helen Zechmeister.

Chapter 1: Dysfunctional Exercise

You need to understand that this is not going to be just another book about "exercise is good for you". We presume you already believe that this is true so we want to dig much deeper into what that means. You probably used to tell your kids to eat their vegetables because they were good for them (and you probably can remember their faces). We also know that as a whole most of you reading this right now don't get excited about exercise, don't live to exercise and can probably list 20 things you would rather be doing. But you also know deep down inside that those 20 things you would rather be doing, you can do better if you have more strength, more endurance, more balance, and more energy. So, we believe it is critical that your exercise program be well thought out and well conceived to support all those things you are really passionate about doing…..for the rest of your life. We believe that many "older adult" or "senior" fitness programs are simply not well designed and are often rather dysfunctional with respect to the human aging process. At our core we believe that we have a lot of control over how we age and the right kinds of exercise can make a huge difference.

As experts in aging and fitness, we know the amazing potential that you hold within you. Potential that can be unleashed with the proper prodding. This is the program that can tap into that potential. We know it works because we have seen the incredible results with hundreds of our own clients that have improved their life dramatically by improving their functional fitness. If you follow this program, we are confident that you will experience the same kind of amazing results that our clients have.

Improve your "doability" (aka functional ability). We call this "doability" because you will be able to do the things you already do even better. Your ability to clean the house, work in the yard, hike a mountain trail, hit a tennis ball, ski down a mountain or carry luggage with greater ease and less discomfort will improve. Plus you will hit the tennis ball harder, ski longer and carry heavier luggage. This program will provide the strength, energy, stamina and flexibility necessary for all of life's tasks. You will even find yourself doing things you haven't done in years because you couldn't do them anymore or trying new things you never thought you could do "at your age".

Feel Better. This improvement in function is accompanied by a reduction in discomfort and pain associated with many physical activities. Participants typically report that minor irritations such as knee pain from osteoarthritis or low back pain get better. Climbing stairs doesn't hurt as much. Working in the garden doesn't come with such high a price as before.

Power the Mind. The neuroscience research from the past 10 years has made it very clear that a person's mind can improve at any age. Exercise and a healthy diet are two major factors that are important to having a healthy brain. Plus having a fit and capable body will boost your self-confidence.

Build Muscle. Although it is not a traditional muscle-building program it will still improve your lean body mass. You will gain muscle (without being bulky at all) and lose body fat creating a leaner and toned body. However, the muscle gain is spread out throughout different parts of the body and includes both the primary and secondary muscle groups. Since this program uses so many muscles in so many different ways the muscle growth is more natural. Instead of looking like a weight lifter or body builder you will just look fit. But maybe more importantly you will be stronger in a functional way. Muscles can get stronger without getting bigger and this program takes advantage of that process so that you get stronger without betting muscle-bound.

Less Injury. "Boomeritis" is a term coined by Dr. Nicholas A. DiNubile, an orthopedic surgeon, in 1999 when trying to explain the explosion in joint and muscle problems by people in their 40's and 50's. When aging joints meet traditional exercise programs the result is often injury and/or pain. The (NGO) Never Grow Old program helps to prevent injury that can occur from exercise, sport, work or daily activities because it helps to improve the accuracy and efficiency of human movement rather than just focusing on building a particular muscle. A leaner, more coordinated, balanced body means less chance of an injury occurring.

Better Balance. Better balance is a great additional benefit to this program. By including a wide variety of stances and body positions, in addition to movements that specifically challenge gait, balance improves significantly. This means a reduced risk of falling and a greater ability to tackle activities that require good balance.

Mr. President

Star college athlete turned actor and past-president Ronald Reagan was a larger-than-life leader. His even and soft-spoken yet appropriately firm style guided a nation through many difficult times such as… He seemed to be able to weather any storm and stand up to any threat during his two terms of office. The "Teflon" president not only came out of political mud-slinging clean as a whistle, but even survived a gunshot wound during an assassination attempt. Nothing, it seemed, could take this great man down. So it was with a mixture of shock, dismay, and sadness that I heard of his diagnosis of Alzheimer's disease. I, and a nation, watched on as gradually, his world began to shrink. He once travelled the globe to speak with the world's most powerful leaders, but eventually could not even communicate with his beloved wife Nancy. We all hate to see such a vibrant and successful person succumb to such a cruel process. To lose the ability to recognize loved ones, communicate with them and take care of one's self. To become a physical and emotional burden on the ones we care about most deeply. And we all fear that we might be next. After all, if it could happen to such a great man as Ronald Reagan, then surely it can happen to me too.

Exercise is a powerful stimulus that can keep you fit, healthy, strong, independent, vibrant, engaged and functional well into late-life. Exercise may add years to your life but, more importantly, it will add life to your years. And it is never too late to start. No matter how many years you have in the rearview mirror you still have many more down the road in front of you, and you want those years to be the best that they can possibly be. After all, you've paid your dues (and your taxes), learned your lessons, worked hard, climbed the ladder, raised children, and given of yourself. And you want to keep doing all of those things you still enjoy and even try some things you've always wanted to do, but just couldn't find the time to fit it in. So you now stand at the pinnacle of life looking over the precipice at a new adventure. Your mind and your spirit are up for the challenge, but you wonder if your body can handle it. You don't quite have the pep in your step that you used to. There are a few more aches and pains in the joints. Some of the tasks that used to be easy as pie are now a little more difficult for your or you may be avoiding them altogether. The aging process is taking its toll. Combine the aging process with years of inactivity (or lack of exercise) and the effects are magnified.

A middle-aged client of ours was concerned about an upcoming trip that she and her husband were taking. They were going on a National Geographic trip to Antarctica. A bucket list trip of a lifetime to be sure. The excursions from the main boat though had our client a little concerned. This involved riding a small rubber boat to one of the little islands and running it up onto the rock beach so everyone could jump out before the water pulled them back into the ocean. If you aren't familiar with this type of boat let me describe it to you. It is an inflatable boat similar to a whitewater raft with large tubular sides. They aren't so easy to climb out of quickly, especially when you are under 5 feet tall like her. Although she was very excited about this adventure she was also extremely worried. What if she couldn't get out of the boat? What if she fell and hurt herself? What if she completely embarrassed herself and her husband? All of these thoughts were swirling through her mind and made her question whether or not she should even try it at all. You can probably identify with her.

There are things you want to do but wonder if your body will allow you to. Whether it's climbing the Temple of the Sun at Machu Picchu, enjoying a bike tour in Holland, spending a day at the zoo with your grandchildren, dancing the night away to your favorite music or simply taking care of your garden, your body needs to be ready for the challenge. Our client learned the power of the exercise system we use. Dan trained her for several months before the trip working specifically on her functional fitness and using the principles and methods that are outlined in this book. She excitedly reported back to us that she not only avoided injury and embarrassment, but she leapt easily out of the boat onto the rocky ground much easier than others 10 years younger than her. Wow was she proud and we were proud for her.

There is a lot of bad information about exercise being passed around today especially when it comes to mature adults. I am fortunate that I have a greater degree of training, education, experience and expertise than most fitness professionals, so I am able to spot bad advice. However, the unsuspecting public is not. I cringe when I see "expert trainers" on TV shows dispensing advice that is just awful at worst and misinformed at best. What makes them an expert anyway? Is it merely the fact that they are on TV or have trained a celebrity? Here are two of my greatest personal biases:
"Senior" exercise

- The fitness programs - These usually have catchy little names with silver, gold, or prime in the titles, but they all reinforce the same myth that once you are older you can't or shouldn't do anything that is challenging or vigorous. So they usually end up spending most of their time exercising while sitting down in a chair or stretching. The exercises are "gentle" and focus on range of motion – neither of which is shown in the research literature to be of much value. I speak to a lot of trainers in different areas of the country and they like to tell me about some "older" client of theirs who can keep up with their younger clients and how amazed they are at their abilities. Really? Is it that surprising that someone who is older is fit and energetic? It's not to me.
- Modifications – I have read most textbooks on exercise for older adults and all of the major certifications for trainers that prepare them to work

with older adults and there is a common theme – modifications. They teach trainers how to take a standard exercise for younger adults and modify it for an older adult. There are two major problems with this. For one, the assumption that they cannot do the exercise "as-is" is ageist (discrimination based on age). Age is definitely not the issue here. I've worked with 40 year olds who need modifications and 80 year olds that do not. Secondly, the assumption is that older adults just need an easier version of the same exercises as young adults. Mature adults are at a different stage of life, facing different challenges and all-around have different needs. Therefore, the exercise program for them should NOT be the same as young adults (an issue which I will explain in more detail later on).

- "Buzz" Words – Oh how the fitness industry loves its buzz words to signify the latest hot trends. There has been metabolic training, core training, mind-body exercise, corrective exercise and now functional training (just to name a few). These exercise methods get hot, trainers and people catch on to them and start following along, but seldom do either have a very good understanding of why they are doing what they are doing. I've seen time and time again where trainers flock to a presentation by an "expert" at a conference to learn one of these latest and greatest methods, and I end up leaving most of them after realizing the "expert" doesn't really know what they are talking about. They are simply repeating words and phrases that they learned from someone else. In fact, early in my career I asked one popular presenter why she spoke on so many different topics. She answered that when asked to give a presentation she always says yes no matter what the topic because she has time to learn about it and prepare her talk. That doesn't make a lot of sense to me. While this book focuses on functional training, you can be assured that we have a very firm grasp about what that means and how to accomplish it. We have spent thousands of hours investigating, learning, reading, experimenting and training in order to accomplish a deep level of expertise.

The fitness programs that many older adults follow are primarily designed to improve muscle size and strength. For better or worse most popular exercise techniques come from the world of bodybuilding in which bigger muscles are the top priority. There is nothing wrong with bodybuilding, but ask yourself, "Do I want to have bulging biceps, a huge back and no neck?" Also, our youth-centric culture dictates to us that these aesthetic characteristics are of utmost importance so the vast majority of exercise facilities and gyms are built from this bodybuilding model. The fitness industry has been doggedly slow in realizing that the 50+ population is not only huge (and growing exponentially) but also has different priorities and needs. Therefore, the industry continues to teach fitness programs to clients as if they were all aspiring to be Arnold Schwarzenegger.

One reason for this is that there is a common misunderstanding of the relationship between muscle strength and physical function. If you asked most fitness professionals today about this topic, I am confident that most of them would say without a doubt that the way to increase physical function (aka "doability") is to increase muscle strength. We will discuss this topic in more detail later on and you will see that this relationship is a little more complicated than that and not quite so simplistic. This is why our passion is to educate mature adults and fitness professionals alike about how to train properly so that physical function is increased.

How Things Went So Wrong

Resistance training is an essential fitness program element and it is doubly important for mature adults. One of the primary challenges of the aging process is the natural loss of muscle mass and strength (a process called sarcopenia) that is magnified by an inactive lifestyle. So consider this: Following traditional progressive resistance training the muscular strength of older adults can increase anywhere from 25% to more than 100% depending on the exercise program being used, the duration of the training, age and gender of the client, and the specific muscle groups being trained. A landmark study by Fiatarone and Singh in the early 1990's showed that heavy resistance training for even 90-100 year olds was safe and effective at improving muscle mass and strength. The following years showed a significant increase in the number of research studies evaluating the effects of resistance exercise with older populations. It has now been very well-established that progressive resistance training can significantly improve muscle mass and strength in adults of all ages. Because of all of this data, it is now typically recommended that mature adults engage in at least 2 days per week of moderate intensity strength training that includes 8-10 exercises involving the major muscle groups using 1-3 sets of 8-12 repetitions each. This is the traditional model.

Following these recommendations, it is common to see mature adults following a basic strengthening program 2-3 days per week using primarily machines. Mature adults can safely and effectively use a wide variety of resistance training methods and equipment such as resistance machines, resistance bands, free weights, body weight, hydraulic and pneumatic equipment. Each has its advantages and disadvantages and it is a misconception that mature adults should only use light dumbbells or easy resistance bands because they might become injured. The muscles of older adults need to be challenged in order to grow (this also known as the overload principle) just as the muscles of younger adults do. Although there may be more orthopedic concerns, resistance exercise has been shown to be generally safe.

The Many older adults use weight-lifting machines that are common in most gyms. The advantages of using machines are that they are pretty easy to use, somewhat "dummy" proof, and isolate the muscle group that is being worked. It is this idea of muscle isolation that is so effective in the world of bodybuilding and has embedded itself into the larger world of fitness. The point is to get into a contraption (typically in a seated position) that places almost all of the work on the targeted muscle and allows the rest of the body to relax. Since that one muscle is doing all of the work then it is going to increase its size and strength quicker. And guess what? It works. If your goal is to improve the size and strength of one particular muscle group then this is a great way to do it. It is this type of muscle isolation program that has been used in many exercise studies with mature adults.

Exercise philosophies and methods for mature adults have come a long way in the past several decades. As more and more data (discussed above) regarding how well resistance training combats sarcopenia (the loss of muscle mass and strength with advancing age) this became the focus of most fitness programs. More recently, though, there has been a shift towards evaluating the functional effects of resistance exercise and the evidence is quite surprising. Startling in fact!

"You missed it by that much!" – Maxwell Smart

Key studies published in 2001, 2004 and 2008 critically evaluated the relationship between the improvement of factors such as strength, joint range of motion, aerobic capacity, body composition, etc. following training with measures of function such as gait speed, chair rise time, stair climbing, balance and weighted lifting tasks. They all concluded the same thing – the relationship is not nearly as strong as what we always assumed it to be. One group of authors (2001) specifically noted that subjects who improved the most on the strength were not necessarily the ones who improved the most on the functional measures. Another group of authors (2004) concluded that strength gains do not equate to similar functional gains. More recently, an extensive review of the literature (Orr et al. 2008) determined that there is limited evidence to show that *progressive resistance training as a single intervention is able to improve balance performance in older adults.*

I don't want you to miss the impact of what this tells us. It is hard for some people to swallow, but the evidence is pretty clear: Stronger is not always better! Traditional muscle-isolation type resistance exercise programs will significantly improve strength but will probably NOT significantly improve physical function. Therefore, a new approach to exercise is needed for mature adults.

The philosophies, principles, strategies and techniques that are used in the Never Grow Old Exercise Program are the keys to improving physical function. We have spent years analyzing the most current research; sharing ideas with the most prominent experts in the field; and training hundreds of clients. We want you to get the same kinds of amazing results that our personal clients have. It is critical that you read, understand and put these principles into action. These principles focus primarily on functional resistance exercise movements but will include some key information on cardiovascular and flexibility exercise as well. From there we will show you different exercise movements that are based on these core principles including pictures and instructions to help guide you. Finally, we provide some sample programming to help you be able to build the program that will best suit your needs given your current level of physical ability.

The program includes three primary components that are to be used together: Functional Warm-Up, Functional Fitness Workouts, and HIIT Cardio. There are 3 levels of the Functional Fitness Workouts that are progressively more challenging. This allows you to select the one that best meets your current level of physical ability and to keep challenging yourself as your functional fitness improves. Keep in mind if you want a video component for your exercise program we have that available at our online fitness program and companion DVD at functionalfitnesssolution.com.

If you want to start moving better, feeling better and looking better, then this is the program for you. Whether you are new to fitness or have been exercising your whole life you will discover an approach to exercise vastly different than what you will see in 95% of the gyms out there. That's because you will now understand how to train your body to get the result that are relevant for you now and will help prepare you to remain functional as you get older. And, by the way, don't think that you won't get stronger with this program because you will. But you will develop functional strength that is useful for life rather than isolated muscle strength which is useful for show.

Let's get started!

Chapter Take-Aways:

How you Train is how you gain.
To maximize your Progress, your exercise program must be progressive in nature.
While traditional strength (resistance) training has been demonstrated to improve strength it has not been shown to improve balance and functional performance.
This book is filled with a philosophy about aging and human function that is based on scientific research, and is not just another exercise book for "seniors".

Never Grow Old!

Chapter 2: The Never Grow Old Functional Fitness Formula

This program is much more than just a bunch of exercises. It is a formula and one that we have spent years and years creating, testing and refining. We have drawn heavily from the most recent functional training research as well as our own expertise in aging to develop highly effective strategies and techniques. We have been able to try out these techniques on hundreds of clients in our living laboratory...our personal training studio. The result is a proven system of training that is incredibly effective, efficient and safe.

The 4 Cornerstones

Any credible system must have a strong foundation. NGO has four cornerstones that together form an incredibly stable foundation for the rest of the program. Each of these alone is good but when joined together they create an incredible synergy that magnifies their impact. Briefly they are:

1.   An in-depth UNDERSTANDING of the aging process and its implications for exercise.
2.   A RECOGNITION of the desires, goals and aspirations that accompany the third age.
3.   A strong BELIEF that people can be fit, healthy, vibrant and functional at any age.
4.   An APPROACH to exercise that is grounded in evidence and honed with experience.

The 2 Pillars

The foundation supports two key pillars that form the core of the NGO system and which many programs miss entirely. These pillars are the concepts of specificity and progressive overload. A good understanding of these concepts will enable you to get the most out of the program.

The Pillar of Specificity states that how a person trains determines the type of gains they make. As I like to tell my students, "How you train is how you gain". In other words, the kinds of exercises that a person performs, and how they perform them will determine the type and magnitude of results that the person sees. This principle is obvious when we consider someone who starts a walking program because they want to improve the strength of their arms. Even to the untrained eye this doesn't make sense. Walking may be a good choice for improving cardiovascular endurance and decreasing health risk but it has virtually no impact at all on arm strength. It is the wrong type of program for the desired results.

Most mature adults would say that one of the most important results that they would like to get from exercise is increased physical function. They want to be able to move better and easier with less discomfort and pain. Whether that means playing golf or tennis, traveling, enjoying hobbies, playing with grandchildren, performing yard work, or whatever it is that is important and enjoyable to them. You probably have similar goals. This program is focused very specifically on increasing physical function. Therefore, every technique, every method, every exercise has been included so that you get to that goal.

Unfortunately, the vast majority of older adults are following programs that have little, if anything, to do with moving better. They are not following the important core principle of specificity and are therefore not getting the biggest functional bang for their exercise buck that they could. This leads many people to become disenchanted or frustrated with exercise because if they can't get the results that are important to them, then why bother exercising in the first place?

The Pillar of Progressive Overload states that the body must continually be challenged with more difficult tasks or exercises in order for it to continue to adapt and grow. The body will adapt only to the level of challenge that you give it and will not improve any more until it is given a greater challenge. There are lots of ways to progressively overload the body such as lifting heavier weights, completing more repetitions, performing the exercise for a longer period of time (e.g. jogging for 30 minutes instead of 20), increasing the intensity, or making a movement more complex. This program uses a myriad of methods, many of which you will rarely see used by even "expert" trainers, to continually overload the body's systems so that you continue to make improvements.

I have worked with hundreds of clients who have missed this principle completely. They either think that what they are doing is "good enough" for a person their age or believe that working out harder will be dangerous for them. I don't know how many times I have followed up with a client or member that has been working out for several months only to find out that they haven't changed their program at all since day one. Their program was kind of tough the first couple weeks and then it became pretty easy after that because their body adapted. Sometimes this can go on for years or even decades.

A Solid Structure: The Seven Key Principles

The final part to the NGO formula is comprised of 7 key principles. These principles have been distilled from hundreds of research studies. I originally developed the principles to help educate fitness professionals how to work more effectively with their middle-aged and older clients. My work has been published in a prominent fitness journals and I have taught these principles to hundreds of fitness professionals at a number of national and international conferences. We have even founded an organization called the Functional Aging Institute and created a certification for fitness professionals called the Functional Aging Specialist to teach this system to thousands of fitness professionals around the world.

So that you have a better understanding of why we have included the types of exercises that we use in this program I will briefly explain each of these key principles.

The 7 Principles
1. Train ALL components of function
2. Be purposeful
3. Train in all 3 planes
4. Train movements before muscles
5. Stand up, stay up
6. Complicated first, simple last
7. Be safe to be successful

Principle #1: Train All Components of Function

There is a long list of variables that contribute to physical function (some of them listed below) and muscle strength is only one of these components. All of these variables are important to the successful completion of functional tasks such as walking, stepping, bending, reaching, lifting, etc. because physical movement is quite complicated. Even the seemingly simple act of walking requires the contribution of around 200 different muscles each playing their part, great or small, to accomplish this task. The program purposefully challenges many of these within a single workout and oftentimes within a single exercise movement. This gives you a lot of "bang for your buck" out of each and every session.

Functional Components (not exhaustive)
- Muscle Strength: How much force the muscle can produce with a single contraction. Typically, this is called one-repetition maximum strength.
- Concentric: A type of muscle contraction in which the muscle shortens and "pulls" two bones closer together. For example, during the lift of a bicep curl the biceps muscle shortens to bring the forearm closer to the upper arm.

- Eccentric: A type of muscle contraction in which the muscle lengthens and allows two bones to move further away from one another. For example, during the "down" phase of the bicep curl the biceps muscle lengthens to allow the forearm to lower away from the upper arm.
- Isometric: A type of muscle contraction in which no length change or movement occurs. For example, if you stop moving your arm in the middle of the bicep curl then the biceps muscle holds its contraction and neither lengthens nor shortens.
- Muscle Endurance: The ability of a muscle to perform repeated contractions over time.
- Muscle Power: The ability of a muscle to produce force quickly. It is the product of force and velocity and is also referred to as explosive strength.
- Contraction Velocity: The ability of a muscle to contract quickly.
- Mobility: The ability to move your body from place to place despite obstacles.
- Normal Gait: The ability to walk in a "normal" manner.
- Joint Flexibility: The ability of a joint to move through its full range of motion.
- Agility: Also called dynamic balance it is the ability to nimbly negotiate obstacles and challenges to balance while moving.
  - Coordination: The ability to use different parts of the body together smoothly and efficiently.
- Postural Control: The ability to sustain the necessary posture to carry out a specific task.
- Somatosensation: The ability to feel sensations of touch, pressure and pain.
- Proprioception: The ability to "know" where your limb is in space and at what angle a joint is without looking. Proprioception is critical during complex activities and those that involve walking or stepping on unstable surfaces.

- Balance: The ability to keep the center of gravity of the body over the base of support. During standing the base of support is the feet. During sitting the base of support becomes the bottom and both feet.

As we age all of these components are affected to some degree. Muscle coordination decreases. Balance worsens. Agility declines. Strength and power decrease. And the list goes on. The reality of function is that training more of these components will lead to better functional outcomes than training fewer components. And this logic is supported by an increasing amount of evidence for the superiority of functional programs compared to traditional strength training programs.

These functional programs typically focus more on the replication of daily tasks with a much greater emphasis on including a broader range of functional components. Special attention is often given to challenging motor control and coordination. Functional task challenges are accomplished by using whole-body movements, often with environmental manipulations, and few, if any, traditional isolation-type exercises.

Principle # 2: Be purposeful.

The Man with No Name

Is anyone cooler than Clint Eastwood? If I were alone on an island and could only choose one actor's film collection to keep me entertained it would be Clint hands-down. I can fondly recall spending hours upon hours watching Clint as the Man with No Name, Dirty Harry and Philo Beddoe (from a couple of my personal childhood favorites Every Which Way But Loose and Any Which Way You Can) in my downstairs rec room. He has been one of my heroes for a long time. In almost all of his films, and especially the spaghetti westerns, Clint is a no-nonsense, straight-to-the-point kind of guy and this seems to be natural for him. When you look at his brief stint as Mayor of Carmel you see this attitude at work…he got things done and did them well. I believe that if Clint Eastwood were a personal trainer he and I would get along marvelously because I believe the same no-nonsense, straight-to-the-point approach is what sets apart great exercise programs from good ones. I often stress with my students and trainers I am teaching that at any point they should be able to answer the question "Why are you doing that particular exercise for that particular client at this point in their training program?" There should be a solid purpose for every exercise movement and every variation that is used and, if not, it needs to be re-evaluated.

You have a limited amount of time and energy to devote to an exercise program so every exercise should have a specific purpose. You don't want to waste your time performing exercises that have minimal value in helping you accomplish your goals. However, the myth of the well-rounded routine is entrenched in our minds. The myth states that a good routine is one that is well-balanced and includes exercises for "every major muscle group." But the best routines are not balanced…they are prioritized. We've trained many individuals that have great leg strength and really don't need much, if any, work in that area. Older men with a background in carpentry, gardening or a related area typically have very strong forearms and arms. Those that are or were significantly overweight often have very strong calf muscles. And the list goes on. Think about it. Wouldn't it make more sense to target the worse areas first before spending time and energy on an area that is doing just fine?

Break away from the constraints of the well-rounded routine and stop wasting your time and energy by performing exercises that do not serve your individual needs and goals. The mature age group is the most heterogeneous (diverse) of any age group, and brings to the table a tremendous range of functional abilities, chronic disease conditions, experiences, and many other factors. But yet despite this incredible diversity you will still hear professionals professing to know what kind of exercise program is best for older adults. Look around. Are you like everyone else your age? So which ones are these professionals talking about? The 75 year old who can run a marathon or the 60 year old who gets winded walking up the stairs? The 80 year old who has been an active weight-lifter for 50 years or the 65 year old couch potato? This kind of blanket approach is akin to ageism (stereotyping by age) and should be avoided at all costs. The NGO system purposefully puts exercises together in a routine that complement one another and when performed together challenge a wide variety of functional components appropriate for your current level of function and conditioning. Plus you have the flexibility to swap out exercises that you feel might be more appropriate for you.

Principle # 3: Train in all 3 planes.

Life is three-dimensional. You reach, bend, lean, turn, twist, stoop and change directions constantly throughout their day. In essence, you continually face challenges in the front to back, side to side and rotational planes – these are the 3 planes of human movement.

Side to Side Plane: Side to side movement or force. Shuffling sideways, arm raises to the side, side-bending or leg raises to the side (even when you are lying down) are all frontal plane movements. Holding a dumbbell in one hand by your side, while standing, would be an example of a frontal plane force. Although you aren't moving, the dumbbell is trying to pull you over and your muscles have to work to resist that force in the frontal plane.

Front to Back or Back to Front Plane: Frontward or backward movement or force. Walking forward or backward, sit-ups, standing up, arm raises to the front and rowing are all sagittal plane movements. If you were in a standing position and someone was pushing on your chest that would be an example of a front to back plane force because, even though you aren't moving, your muscles have to resist to keep you from falling backwards. If someone were pushing on your back then that would be a back to front plane force.

Rotational Plane: Twisting movement or force. This could be rotating or twisting your upper body while your lower body stays in place or twisting your lower body while your upper body stays in place or moving both (either in the same or opposite directions) simultaneously. It can also include a force that wants you to rotate but that you resist against.

Despite this three-dimensional aspect of life most exercise routines for older adults are very one-dimensional. Several reasons have contributed to this phenomenon:

• We have all been heavily influenced by our body-building roots within the fitness industry. While functional training methods and tools are becoming more popular the majority of the industry still focuses on the aesthetic goals of younger members and clients. This means using machines or free weights to isolate individual muscle groups for maximum hypertrophy, or growth.

• Sarcopenia (age-related loss of muscle mass) is still regarded by many as the primary enemy of function with advancing age. Therefore, if muscle loss is the enemy then the cure must be to maximize muscle mass gains through heavy resistance training using the aforementioned body-building methods and equipment.

• Trainers that work with older clients may not have specialized training for this population and therefore simply transfer what they know about training younger clients to their older clients with some "common sense" modifications. Take, for example, one of our clients Ann. Ann, a slightly overweight but healthy woman in her early 60's, came to our facility after training with another personal trainer whose background was bodybuilding. We quickly discovered that Ann's previous trainer developed a very generic, modified bodybuilding routine for her that had little to do with her individual needs or goals. The modifications including "common sense" strategies such as doing bicep curls in a seated position instead of standing (and with very light weights); performing crunches on an incline bench set at about 45 degrees (so that it assisted her); and incline chest press using very light dumbbells. It was obvious that this trainer had little to no knowledge, skill or experience working with older adults and therefore simply adopted what he did know (bodybuilding).

The multi-dimensional training approach falls in line with the advice of some of the top experts in the field such as Gary Gray, PT and Stuart McGill, PhD who advocate for a lesser focus on traditional strength training methods and a greater focus on multi-planar movements that challenge the body in ways that are more beneficial to functional task performance. The reason the NGO program uses so many different body positions (standing, half-kneeling, kneeling, etc.), arm variations (both arms, one arm, alternating, etc.), movement patterns and equipment is to purposefully challenge the body in different planes.

Principle # 4: Train movements before muscles.

As discussed earlier, traditional strength training exercises offer some benefits for combating sarcopenia (loss of muscle mass due to age,) building strength, and, to a lesser degree, for improving function. So it is difficult to conclude that these exercises are not functional at all. Even arm curls are functional to a certain degree because you have to use your biceps to lift or pull objects. So it is better to view exercises along a functional continuum with some exercises having a more distant relationship to functional performance (e.g. less functional) and others having a closer relationship to functional performance (e.g. more functional). While individual needs must always be considered, the evidence point to the use of multi-dimensional exercises that address multiple components of function as the primary focus of an exercise routine for mature clients. Traditional strength movements that isolate individual muscle groups can be used to supplement the functional exercises when muscle strength is really low in one area of the body.

For example, a person that cannot stand up from a seated position without using their hands is obviously very weak in the legs. They need to practice the functional movement of standing up from a seated position using their arms to assist them as little as possible. But they should also perform some traditional leg strengthening exercises such as seated leg extensions, leg curls and calf raises. The combination of the functional and traditional strength movements will yield the best result. You will quickly find that in the NGO program we utilize a variety of combinations of more functional and less functional movements.

Principle #5: Stand up, Stay up.

Mobility is a critical component for the continued health and longevity of mature adults. Loss of mobility can lead to a downward "death spiral" of declining health and activity levels. We see this all the time when older adults get injured or become sick and have to lay or sit around for several weeks. Their health and function goes downhill quickly because they are so inactive. But beyond that mobility is a critical component of life satisfaction for many mature adults. Loss of mobility usually means loss of independence. People can no longer work, shop, play, or do household chores because they cannot get up and around to do them. Then they end up relying on help from others. Related to this is risk of falling. Falls are a significant threat to the mature population often leading to hospitalization, the need for long-term care and even the leading cause of accidental death. The majority of exercises should be performed in a standing or semi-standing position (e.g. kneeling, half-kneeling, lunge, etc.). Mobility and balance are best improved in standing positions.

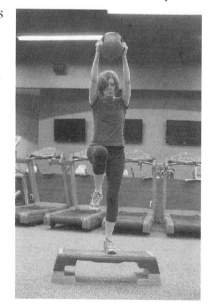

The standing position utilizes many more muscle groups than sitting and is a more complex neuromuscular challenge that requires greater degrees of strength, proprioception, center of gravity control and postural stability. In addition, it is much more difficult to give multi-planar challenges (see Principle #1) while seated. Therefore, seated exercises should be used minimally in a functional exercise routine.

Seated exercise may be purposeful when:
a.	You become fatigued
b.	You are not yet ready for higher-level progressions or you are too unstable on your feet
c.	The movement involves sit-to-stand transitions
d.	You are frail and/or at the lowest end of the functional spectrum (e.g. rehabilitation, nursing homes)

Principle #6: Complicated first, simple last.

During the course of an exercise training session it is typical for energy and focus to wane as both muscle and mental fatigue set in. For mature clients this loss of energy and focus can create potentially dangerous scenarios and increase risk of injury (discussed further in Principle #7). The longer the session continues the more likelihood that attention and performance will wane. You should always be mindful of your level of fatigue and adjust your training session accordingly.

Recognizing the decline in energy and focus it is prudent then to perform more complicated tasks earlier in the session while you are still fresh physically and mentally. More complicated movements include dynamic balance tasks, gait variations, agility drills (ladder, dot, obstacles) and multi-planar movements. The latter parts of the session would be more appropriate for isolated strength training, seated movements and floor work.

Be careful not to confuse complexity with intensity. An isolated strength movement is not complex but it can be very intense depending upon the resistance challenge that is used. So just because a movement is performed closer to the end of the session does not mean that it is easier than ones that occurred earlier

It is important to note that when using unstable surfaces force production capabilities decrease because more energy is required to stabilize the joints. As an example, performing a squat on the floor allows you to direct the majority of forces upwards and maximize the amount of weight lifted. However, when performing a squat on a balance pad, energy is used to keep the knees in alignment and the center of mass over the base of support (feet) so that you cannot lift as much weight.

Principle #7: Be safe to be successful.

Getting off the traditional exercise machines in order to perform standing, dynamic, multi-dimensional exercises of increasing complexity brings with it an increase in risk of falling and injury. Therefore, it is your responsibility to take the appropriate measures to ensure safety while maximizing the potential for success.

First off be honest about your current level of health and physical ability. While we want you to step out of your comfort zone and put as much as you can into your workouts we also want you to be safe. If you have significant health concerns such as cardiovascular disease, joint replacements, diabetes, osteoporosis or similar conditions then modify your program accordingly.

The primary safety concern that needs to be addressed in a functional exercise program is the likelihood of a fall. Many of the movements we use will either rely on good balance (and stability) or will purposefully challenge balance. Position yourself so that you have a chair, table or railing to rely on if you need it and make sure the environment is free of trip hazards.

- Make sure you can perform a movement really well before trying a more complicated variation. Progressions that are implemented too quickly can lead to frustration, failure and, potentially, injury.

Chapter Take Aways:

How you train is how you will gain or improve

In order for your body to respond you must progressively challenge it

Safety always takes precedence when choosing exercise movements

Have a purpose for what you are doing

Chapter 3: The Never Grow Old Program

About the Program

We have developed exercise strategies based on the 4 Cornerstone, the 2 Pillars and the 7 Key Principles for Functional Training, discussed in the previous chapter, to challenge individuals at all levels of fitness and functional ability. Everything has a purpose and this program manipulates variables such as body position, stance, arm position, arm movement patterns, direction, distance, depth, velocity, equipment, and complexity in a purposeful manner in order to create exercise movements that will accomplish our goal of improving physical function (remember the principle of specificity). These exercise movements are then further "tweaked" (by mixing up the variables) in a highly-ordered process to ensure that you are progressively challenged as you improve your functional fitness.

These "tweaks" allow us to create a continuum of functional challenge. We can change just one variable to either bump up the challenge just a little bit or to refocus the exercise movement to work on a different component of function altogether. We can also change multiple variables simultaneously to significantly increase the functional demand. The combinations are almost limitless. This is great news for you because the programs will never get boring or routine! For example, consider how some simple variations in a row movement can alter the demands placed on the core and trunk. We will start with a standing, split-stance (one foot slightly ahead of the other), two-arm row using resistance tubing.

In this position the trunk is being pulled forward creating a large sagittal plane (back to front) demand. This causes the posterior chain muscles (muscles on the back of the body) to really work to keep the body in an upright position.

However, by dropping out the left hand and only using the right hand to perform the row movement we can change the demand on the trunk. Instead of a sagittal plane demand there is now a transverse (rotational) plane demand because only one hand is holding the resistance which creates an imbalance between the right and left sides. Instead of being pulled forward the trunk is pulled into rotation (twisting) which it must resist. This completely changes the muscle activation in the back and hips. We can further increase the challenge by adding a backwards lunge to this movement. So now the person must step backwards with the right leg into a lunge position while simultaneously performing a tubing row with the right hand. Not only does this require a lot more lower-body strength it is also a more complicated movement which requires much more motor control, coordination, and balance to perform.

This is just one simple example of how small and seemingly insignificant changes in the variables of an exercise movement can create important differences in the demands on the body. These manipulations are embedded throughout the program and although we want you to understand the philosophy and approach behind the workouts the great thing is that you don't have to think about it. We've done all of the work for you by creating workouts that are extremely well-balanced and focused.

Below is a summary of some of the progressions that are utilized throughout the program.

General Progressions for Increasing Functional Fitness
From Single Joint to Multi-Joint
From More Stable to Less Stable
From Simple to Complex

From Slower to Faster

From Shorter to Longer

From Static to Dynamic

From Single Plane to Multiple Planes

From Individual Movements to Combinations of Movements

From Lower Resistance to Higher Resistance

From Balanced to Unbalanced

About the Workouts

A complete exercise session consists of first a Dynamic Warm-Up, followed by a Functional Fitness Workout. Each of these components is important and should not be skipped. The warm-ups take about 4 minutes; the workouts about 15-20 minutes, so a total of 20-25 minutes three times per week. That is all it takes to get great results. The Dynamic Warm-Up and the Functional Fitness Workouts can be easily modified to meet your needs. For example, if you have osteoarthritis of the knees then you might need a little longer than 4 minutes to really get the joints ready to go. In that case it would be valuable to walk or ride a stationary bike for 5 minutes before the Dynamic Warm-Up. In addition we encourage you to engage is some functional stretching following your workouts, you may have a stretching routine that you already like and have gotten great results from. If you need additional Functional Flexibility routines please visit our online fitness program at functionalfitnessolution.com. Following the exercise sessions you have the option of performing some light to moderate cardiovascular exercise of your choosing. Since you have the High-Intensity Interval Training program on off-days then these cardio workouts should not be high-intensity. Consider 20-45 minutes of moderate cardio exercise depending on your current level of fitness, goals, and time constraints. Moderate intensity means a rating of 13-15 ("somewhat hard" to "hard") on the Rating of Perceived Exertion (RPE) scale or 65-75% of maximal heart rate (maximal heart rate can be estimated by the equation 220-age). Also, it is wise to vary your mode of exercise: treadmill, walk outside, upright bike, recumbent bike, swim, hike, stepper, recumbent stepper, elliptical, etc. There are many options to choose from so mix it up. Keep it fresh. Keep it interesting.

Two days per week you will be performing a Cardio Warm-Up, High-Intensity Interval Training (HIIT) program, followed by some light stretching. The cardio warm-up can simply be 5-10 minutes of light activity such as walking, stationary biking, jogging, elliptical trainer, etc. The HIIT program will take about 15-20 minutes and is covered in detail elsewhere. The total time is 30-35 minutes. The remaining two days per week should be devoted to rest, relaxation, and any leisure activities you enjoy to recharge your batteries

Functional Fitness Workout

The program has been divided into three levels so that people of all ages and abilities can jump into the program and be challenged appropriately. Choosing the right level for you requires a little bit of trial and error. WE RECOMMEND THAT EVERYONE TRY A LEVEL I WORKOUT FIRST. If the workout is too easy then move up a level and keep doing so until you find a level that appropriately challenges you. So it may take two to three workouts at the most before you find the right level for you.

However, it is WAY better to try a workout that is too easy and then move up than to attempt a workout that is above your capabilities and possibly risk getting injured or sore or aggravating an existing condition. Remember, discretion is the better part of valor. Use the descriptions of the levels below to help you choose where to begin. One point of caution however, we have had many new clients who considered themselves to be fit and who worked out regularly in a gym that thought they could easily jump right into an intermediate or advanced level functional workout. But they were quickly humbled when it wasn't as easy as they thought. They realized that a functional workout is VERY different from a typical gym workout because the whole body is basically working the entire time and muscles they never knew they had are used. So, again, we recommend you start lower and then move up as you need to.

Level I – Beginners

This level is best suited for inactive people who have never exercised or haven't exercised in a while and would consider themselves to have a low overall level of fitness. If you have some difficulty climbing a flight of stairs, performing chores and/or getting down to and up from the floor then this is probably the right level for you. In addition, if you feel like you are more fit than what I've described but exercise intimidates you and you are concerned whether or not you are going to be able to follow along correctly then you should also start here. Even if the exercises themselves are not very difficult you will learn the system and terminology and develop confidence in your own abilities. These exercises are less complicated and focus heavily on developing a basic level of functional strength. Only one set of each exercise is performed and there is an emphasis on performing the movements correctly.

Level II – Intermediate

This is the level that most healthy, active adults would fall into. It is best suited for active folks without any significant health concerns or physical limitations who consider themselves to be relative fit and able-bodied. If you currently exercise regularly performing a variety of free weight movements or follow a strength-based group exercise class then this is the level for you. The exercise movements are more complicated with much more variety in the variables mentioned earlier (stance, direction, arm movement patterns, etc.). In addition, the combinations of movements within the triple-sets are more challenging and the pace is faster with less rest in-between triple-sets.

Level III – Advanced

This is designed for the active person who is an experienced exerciser. If you are fitter than average and ready for a fun, exciting and fast-paced program to improve your functional fitness then Level III is for you. Most exercises are combination movements so that you get the most bang for your buck out of each one. As pointed out earlier, though, performing a functional workout is different than a traditional workout so do not try this level for your first workout even if you think you can handle it.

Equipment

Equipment is kept to a minimum but may include resistance tubing, dumbbells, step (or stair), or an exercise mat. Many exercises only utilize body weight. By keeping equipment to a minimum the workouts become very portable and can be performed almost anywhere. If this equipment is unfamiliar to you then read the descriptions below.

Resistance Tubing: We recommend purchasing two resistance tubes with handles and a door anchor (optional). Resistance tubes can be purchased at almost any sports store, big box store (Walmart, Target) or online retailer for less than $10 each. They should be 5-6' in length and the two tubes should be different resistance levels. The reason for this is that different muscles have different natural strength levels so you want to have at least two different levels of resistance tubing to accommodate them. Most manufacturers have at least four levels of resistance that are color-coded. For each workout the goal is to use as much resistance as possible while still being able to complete the number of repetitions with good form so having a couple options of different resistance levels is essential. You may have a resistance band or two at home from physical therapy sessions that you have done in the past. I encourage you to purchase tubing with handles instead. They are going to be much more comfortable to use than the bands. The door anchor enables you to secure the tubing to a doorjamb and then move it quickly and easily when needed. The exercises in the program may require the tubing to be anchored at ankle level, chest level or even above the head. If you do not have a railing, post, or other heavy object to secure the tubing to then a door anchor is a great option. Plus it can easily travel with you wherever you go (even to a hotel!).

Dumbbells: We recommend that you have at least two different pairs of dumbbells. It is difficult to specify which weight sizes to have available because people vary considerably with what they can use. The weights need to be light/moderate and moderate for your capabilities. For Levels I and II this probably means 5lbs and 10lbs. For Levels III this probably means 10lbs and 20lbs but this could vary. These are pretty inexpensive and, like resistance tubing, can be purchased at many stores. However, if you really want to have lots of options available without purchasing a bunch of different size dumbbells then you could get an adjustable pair of dumbbells. With the slide of a pin or the turn of a dial you can quickly and easily change the weight of the dumbbell. These are typically $150-$200 but are worth the cost.

Step: A 6"-12" stepstool, exercise step or even a stair is acceptable. If it is a stepstool then make sure that it is stable and will not slide or tip over if you step on the edge of it. For Levels I and II the bottom stair of a staircase is a really good height to use. However, for Levels III you will probably want to invest in a taller step of some sort and preferably one that is adjustable. These can also be purchased at any sports store, bit box store or many online retailers (price range varies considerably).

Exercise Mat: If you do not have a soft surface, such as carpeting, to exercise on then an exercise mat would be a great addition. A mat will be especially useful for Levels II and III that incorporate more floor work for the core..

We want you to be successful and get the most benefit out of this program that is possible. These workouts are effective as long as you put in the time, effort and consistency that is required. So we've put together some helpful information for you so that you can do just that.

Functional Movement Terminology
The following terms are used in the description of the exercise movements and during the workout videos. Understanding them is essential to performing the movements properly.

Arm Movement Patterns
Bilateral (In Sync): Using both hands/arms simultaneously. Each hand/arm is moving in the same direction as the other at all times such as the arms during a bench press.

Alternating: Both hands/arms are used but at different times. One hand/arm will perform the movement and then the other hand/arm will perform the movement.

Reciprocating (Out of Sync): Both hands/arms move in opposite directions simultaneously.

Unilateral: Only one hand/arm is used while the other rests or is used for balance.

Bilateral Opposite: One hand pushes or pulls in one direction while the other hand pushes or pulls in the opposite direction. For example, one hand could be performing a row while the other hand is performing a chest press. It can be performed alternating or out-of-sync.

Press: A pushing movement where the limb is moving away from the body against resistance.

Row: This is a pulling movement where the limb is moving towards the body against resistance.

Stances and Body Positions
Shoulder-Width: Standing position where the feet are placed about shoulder-width apart.

Tandem: One foot is placed directly in front of the other as if walking on a line. This can be heel to toe or the front foot can be placed a little ahead of the back foot.

Semi-Tandem: One foot is placed slightly ahead of the other but not directly in front (like in the tandem position). This position is a little easier balance position than the tandem position.

Split-Stance or Lunge: One foot is placed well ahead of the other foot like when taking a large step. The upper body remains erect and upright.

Kneeling: Both knees are on the ground with the body erect and upright. Typically a pad or pillow is placed beneath the knees for comfort.

Half-Kneeling: One knee is placed on the ground and the other foot is placed in front of the body with the body erect and upright. Typically a pad or pillow is placed beneath the knee for comfort.

Quadruped: On hands and knees. Hands are directly beneath the shoulders and knees are directly beneath the hips. Head should remain in line with the spine (look at the floor). Keep back in a neutral position to avoid a "hump" in the upper back or "dip" in the lower back.

How To Use the Resistance Tubing Effectively

Resistance bands and tubes are versatile tools that can challenge even the fittest of individuals if used properly. Following are some important tips for you to consider when using the tubing in your routine.

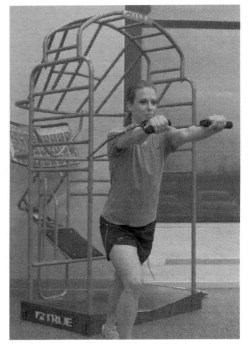

    Tip #1: Anchor Well – Make sure that whatever you attach the tubing to is solid and won't fall over or break when you apply resistance. Using a door anchor in a doorjamb is a great choice but you could also use a support pole or a stair railing as well. Since some movements use either reciprocating or unilateral arm movements then simply looping the band around a pole won't work all of the time. There is a method that will allow you to use all arm movements and quickly adjust the height. Fold the tubing in half and wrap the tubing around the pole or rail.

You should now have both handles in one hand and the folded mid-point of the tubing in the other. Feed the handles through the loop created at the mid-point of the tubing. Pull the handles through completely until the tubing is secured against the pole or rail. Now you can perform all arm movements without having to adjust it.

Tip #2: Move to Adjust Resistance – When performing an exercise movement with tubing you may find that it is either too easy or too difficult. A quick way to adjust the resistance is to either move closer to where it is anchored (making the movement easier) or to move further away from where it is anchored (making the movement more difficult). Make these adjustments quickly and remember that the last few repetitions of each exercise need to be challenging for you or you will not be getting the most benefit out of it.

Tip #3: Control in Both Directions – Since tubing is elastic it tends to "snap back" when you pull it. It is important that you control the movement in both directions. Do not allow it to "snap back" but rather move in slow and controlled movement. When you are done with the exercise don't just let the tubing go if it is still stretched because it will fly around and hit something or possibly someone standing nearby.

Tip #4: Get a New One – At some point the resistance tubing you are using is going to get easier and easier to use (as you get stronger and stronger). Following Tip #2 you can move further and further away in order to increase the resistance level but at some point you will reach the limits of its stretch. It is now time to invest in a new resistance tube that is more challenging. This is a great feeling because you know you have gotten stronger.

How To Use The Dumbbells Effectively

There are several common mistakes that we want to make sure you avoid when using dumbbells in your workouts. Avoiding these errors will ensure that you are being safe with the dumbbells and using them properly in order to get the most benefit out of your program.

Mistake #1: Isaac Newton Would Roll Over in His Grave – Dumbbells are gravity-based equipment. Since gravity pulls objects down to the ground then that means dumbbells need to move in line with the pull of gravity in order to work properly. So any exercise using dumbbells needs to move them primarily up and down (perpendicular to the floor). Any exercise movement that moves the dumbbells parallel to the floor is not using them properly, unless

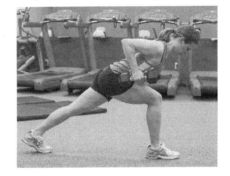

it is primarily for balance or stability training movements. Because dumbbell movements are gravity-based and tubing is not then these two pieces cannot always be swapped out for a particular exercise with the same result. For example, if you are performing a standing row with tubing you cannot substitute dumbbells without also changing your body position. In order to use dumbbells in a rowing movement you would need to lean over so that your trunk is facing the ground. In this position you can use the effects of gravity and make Isaac Newton proud.

Mistake #2: Too Much Swing – When any exercise becomes difficult or when your muscles become tired there is a tendency to "cheat". One of the common cheating movements when using dumbbells is swinging the weights instead of lifting them in a slow and controlled fashion. By swinging the weights into the movement momentum is created which helps you perform the movement but doesn't accomplish the primary goal of working the muscle and increases the risk of accident or injury. Whenever possible using slow and controlled movements with dumbbells. If you cannot complete the number of repetitions with good form then simply drop to a lighter dumbbell in order to finish the set. However, there are some exercise movements using resistance tubing that we will have you do as quickly as possible in order to work on muscle power. Make sure you still use good form when performing these kinds of exercises.

Mistake #3: Easy Cheesy – It is imperative that you use dumbbells that are challenging for you to complete the number of repetitions for a particular movement. In my experience people tend to stick with the same weight for a variety of movements and stay at the same weight even when they could use a heavier one. Different muscle groups are stronger than others and thus require heavier dumbbells. Don't be afraid to use a heavier weight for a particular exercise. One good way to judge that is to honestly ask yourself if you could have completed a couple more repetitions with good form beyond what the set called for. So if you performed a set of 12 repetitions but could have done 2 more with good form then it is time to bump up the weight a little. When performing multiple sets you should ask yourself this question following the last set.

How to customize the workout to meet your needs

These workouts allow for a large degree of customization. The exercise movements can be adjusted or substituted to meet your particular needs, conditions and abilities. We don't want you to shy away from trying new things or getting better at movements that you aren't quite so comfortable with at first but we do want you to make the workouts your own since we cannot be there with you personally to make the adjustments for you. There are many opportunities for you to make adjustments or modifications. Here are just a few suggestions: Don't squat or lunge quite so low. Don't step quite so far. Take rests as you need them. Alter the body or stance position so that you feel more stable. Use a shorter step. Slow down.

Listen to your body and the advice of your medical professionals. I have osteoarthritis in both knees but I exercise regularly (which really helps them to feel better) and I have learned which movements or which types of movements bother them the most. I personally follow the types of workouts you see in Level 3 and I am in my 40's. They make me feel so much better and are so much easier on my knees than traditional exercises although I still include several traditional exercises (mainly just for looks) as supplements to my functional fitness program. So don't be afraid to use your own discretion about what you can do.

Before You Begin
Environment: There needs to be enough room (8'x8' or larger) for you to move around in freely, something to anchor your tubing to and a stair nearby if you don't have an exercise step. It should be free of any clutter, electrical cords and other trip hazards. Secure rugs to the floor and have a wall or sturdy table/chair nearby to use as a balance aid if needed.

Clothing: Use non-slip and preferably athletic shoes. No flats, heels, sandals, flip-flops or slides. You may exercise barefoot if you prefer. Wear athletic or comfortable clothing that allows complete freedom of movement and allows you to stay cool.

Signs and Symptoms: If you experience any of the following signs or symptoms during your workout then stop and seek medical attention:

- Dizziness
- Nausea
- Unusual shortness of breath
- Chest pain or tightness
- Pain in neck or jaw or radiating down the left arm
- Lightheadedness

Energy: Perform workouts only when you are well-fueled, well hydrated and well rested. Have a water bottle handy to sip on during and after your workout.

Chapter Take Aways:

Functional Workouts may be different from exercise routines you are accustomed to, and may be more challenging than they appear.
Progress appropriately, start easy and move to more challenging when ready.
Be sure to properly warm-up.
To find video versions of our workouts visit our website:
www.functionalfitnesssolution.com

Never Grow Old!

Chapter 4: Functional Fitness Workouts

This chapter will be exercises demonstrated by several different models. Our Models are four clients in their 40s, 50s, 70s and 80s and two of our trainers one in her 30s and one in her 40s. They will be demonstrating a wide range of exercise movements from beginner to advanced. You will want to use this chapter in combination with Chapter 5, as well as our online video library where we display numerous exercises in live video form so you can see the movement in action. Keep in mind some of the beginner exercises may be easy for you and others may be very challenging. We encourage you to begin with both beginner routines and if those prove to be easy, then progress to the intermediate routines. However if you are challenged by some of the beginner exercises we encourage you to repeat those for a few weeks, before progressing to the intermediate routines. All of the exercises are designed to be performed with 1 set of 12-15 repetitions per exercise. To increase the challenge you can add a 2nd set, or perform the routine a 2nd time through. Additionally you could increase the resistance being used if it requires a weight. Finally another way to make the workouts more challenging is to shorten your rest in between each exercise, so you are moving from exercise to exercise as continuously as possible without rest breaks. We believe this collection of exercise demonstrations is one of the more comprehensive showing models over the age of 70 and 80. We hope this will be a helpful resource for you to continue to add new and challenging exercise movements to your regimen. We strongly encourage you to use our Resource pages listed in the back of the book so you can see all of these and more demonstrated in person in video. And of course check back often at our companion website functionalfitnesssolution.com. Seeing the exercise movements demonstrated in action will help you even more be sure to perform them correctly. You may also want to seek out the guidance of a fitness professional in your area to help you with ensuring proper form. Since Safety is one of our Principles of training it is extremely important to us that you perform any and all exercises displayed here in a safe and correct manner.

We believe it is always important to warm-up to prepare your body for exercise. If you already have a warm-up routine you know works for all your joints and muscles you may continue to use that provided it thoroughly prepares you for strength training your entire body. We are providing a functional warm-up routine first which you can use before any of the exercise routines. As you advance you may want to use the Beginner workouts as your warm-up routine.

Functional Warm Up

WoodChops using a 4-6 lbs weight. We picture it with a Corball (medicine ball with handles) but you could use a medicine ball or even a dumbbell. You want to move the object from over one shoulder to outside one foot as if you are moving in a diagonal chopping motion

Marching, As it implies raising your knees high as you walk across a room or hallway

Straddle March/Walk You can perform this both walking or marching pretend as if you are straddling a log on the ground

Total Body Extensions, similar to a Jump Squat you are Squatting/Reaching down to touch the floor or your feet and then extending overhead as high as you can and up on your tip toes, without leaving the floor.

Side to Side Rotations, we picture this with a Corball, but you could use a dumbbell or start with no weight at all. Shift your weight from side to side and rotate about the waist.

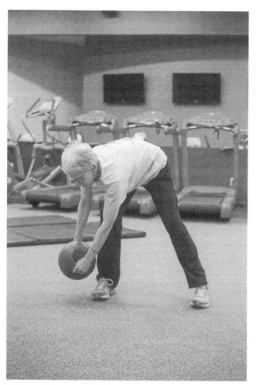

Woodchops (a)

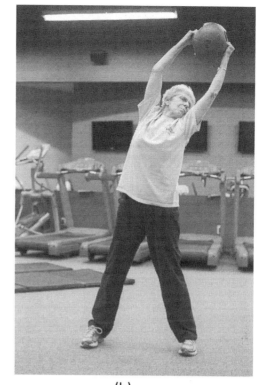

(b)

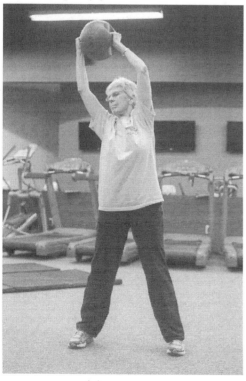

(c)

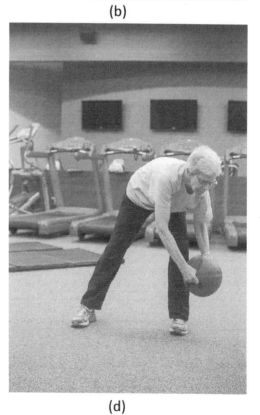

(d)

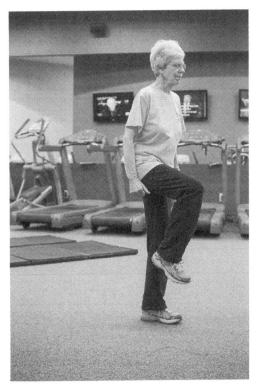 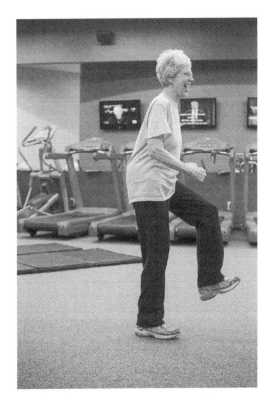

Marching

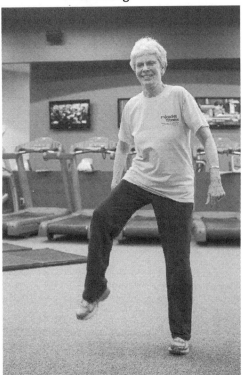 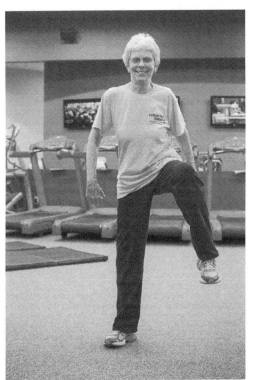

Straddle March/Walk

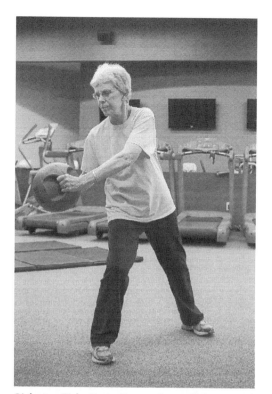 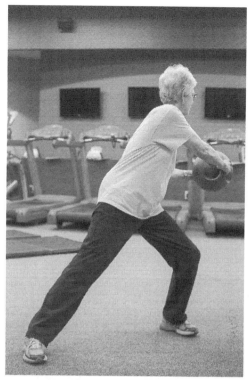

Side to Side Rotations, Step Side to Side Shifting your Weight and Rotating

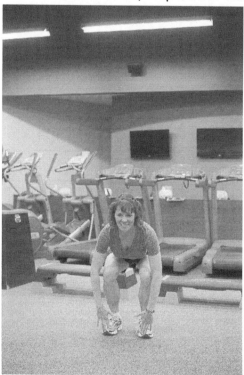 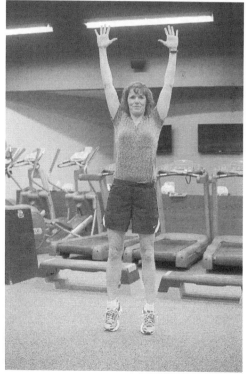

Total Body Extension, Squat Down touch the floor/feet and extend overhead

Beginner Routine #1

Chair Stands: At the beginner level you can use your hands as much as needed

Stepping Over a Dog or Parking Block: As it sounds in all directions, forwards, backwards, sideways.

Mini-Lunges

Bridge: Lying on Mat, feet flat on Mat, Raise your Hips/Butt

Pushups on your knees: Modification if you can't get on the floor you can use a wall or bench

Tandem Walking: Walking as if on a balance beam, one foot in front of the other

One Arm Cable Punch/Press

Bent Over Row in a lunge stance one arm

Total Body Extensions (Squat Jump, no jump)

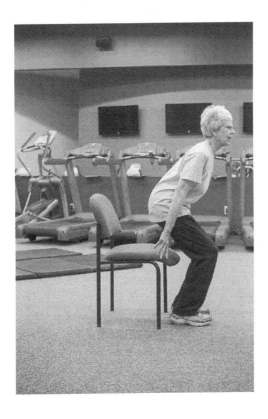 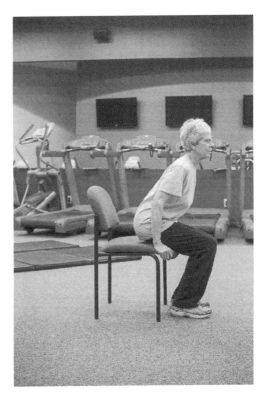

Chair Stands   (a)   (b)

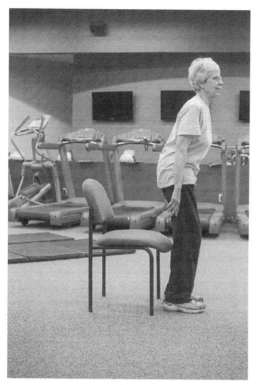

(c)

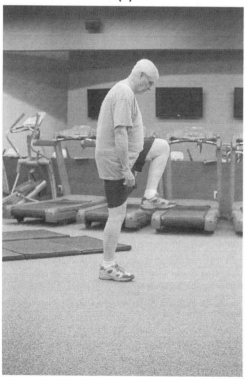

Stepping over an object(a)

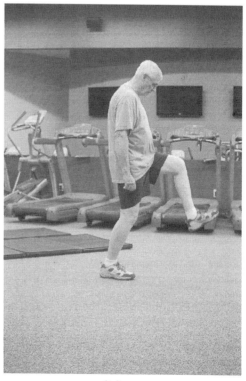

(b)

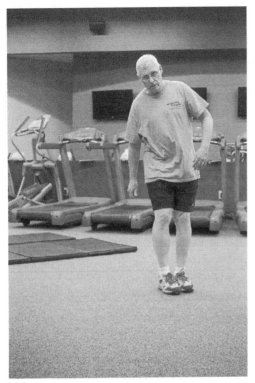 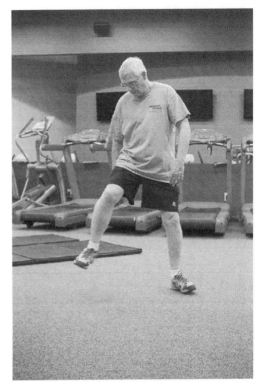

Stepping sideways (a)   (b)

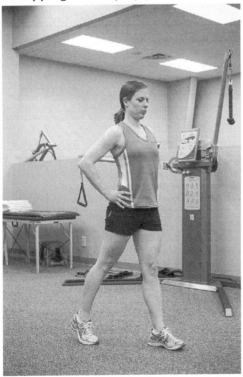 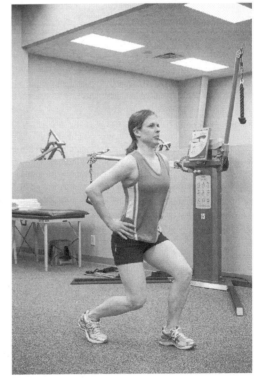

Mini Lunges (a)   (b)

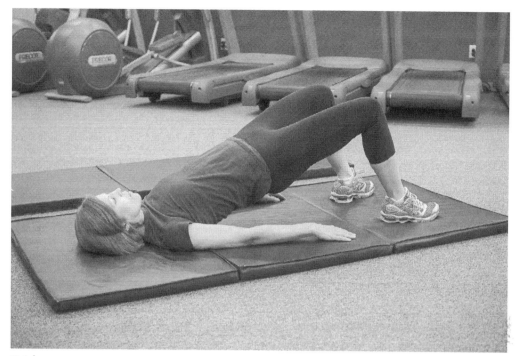

Bridge

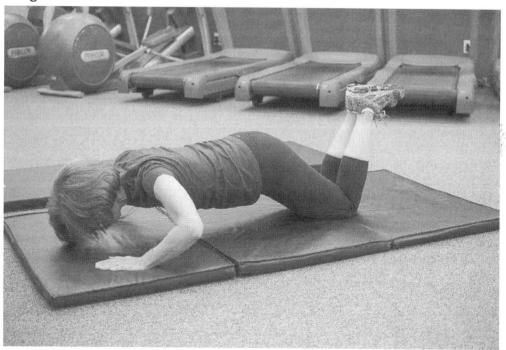

Modified Pushups on Knees (a)

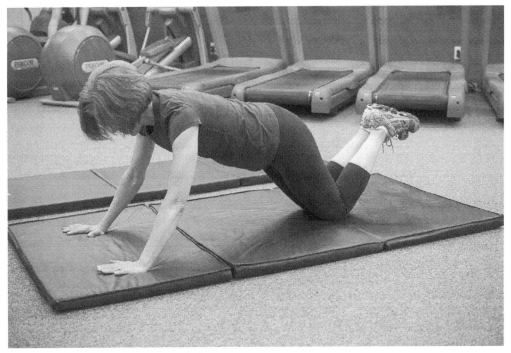

Modified Pushups on Knees (b)

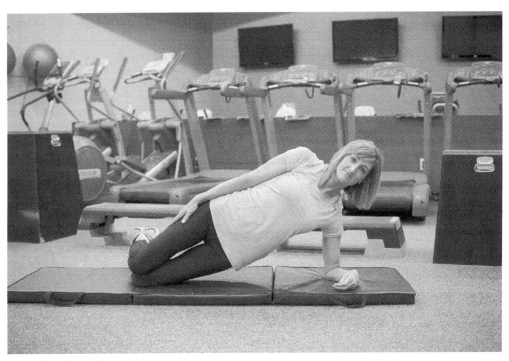

Side Plank on Knees

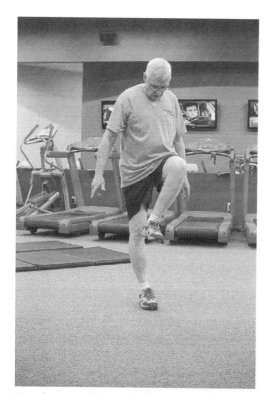
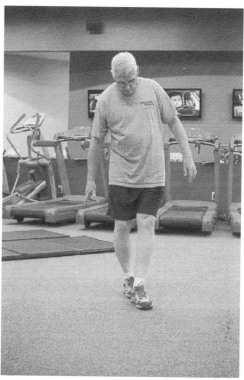

Tandem walking, Walking one foot directly in front of the other

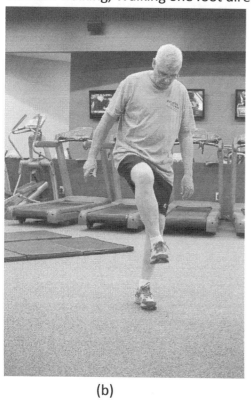
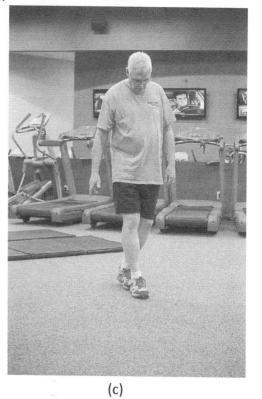

(b)

(c)

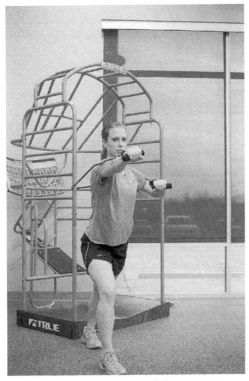

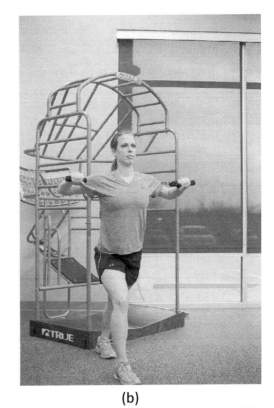

One Arm Cable Punch (a)

(b)

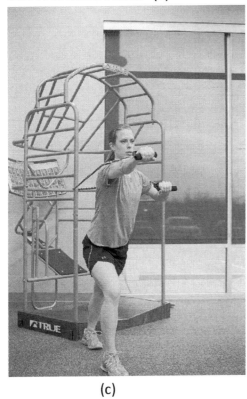

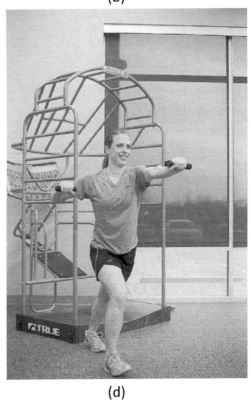

(c)

(d)

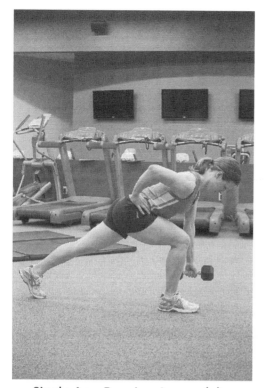

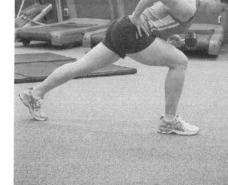

Single Arm Row in a Lunge (a)

(b)

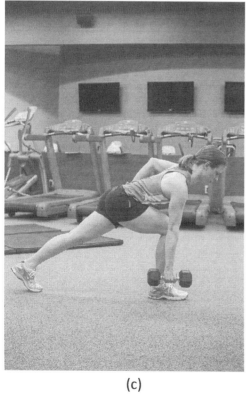

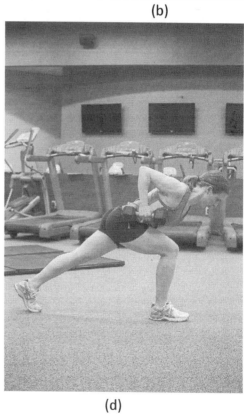

(c)

(d)

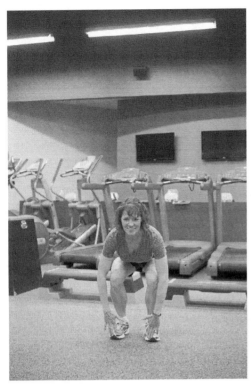 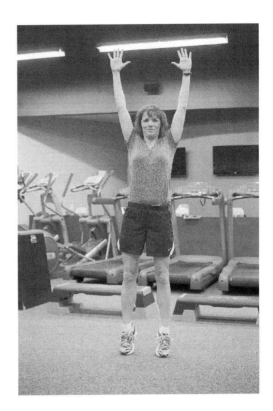

Total Body Extensions

Beginner routine number 2

Chair Stands (with arms crossed)

Lunge Stance (Big Step) with Crossover Reach: Using Dumbbells take a large step and hold that position and crossover right and left with dumbbells after 12-15 reps switch feet and repeat

Tandem Walking: Walking a Straight line same as in routine #1

Shrugs: Hold Dumbbells at your side and raise your shoulders (shrug them)

Walking on Heels   (be careful this is harder than it looks)

Step-Ups   Using a step simply step up and down.

Lunges

Plank

Lunge Stance Arm Curls

Squats

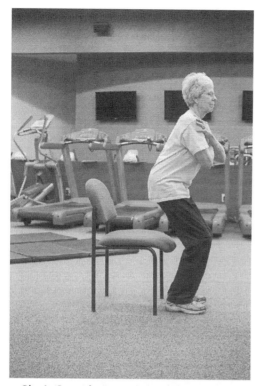 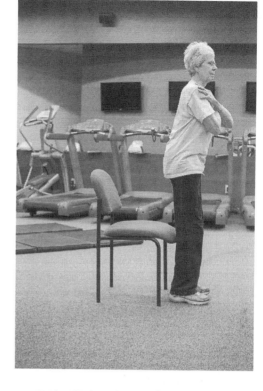

Chair Stands Arm Crossed

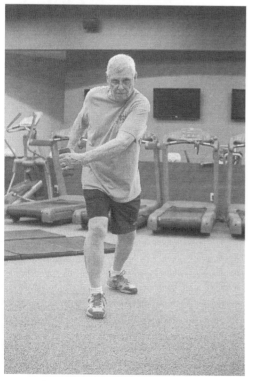 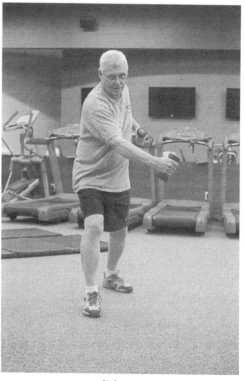

Lunge Stance Crossover Reach

(b)

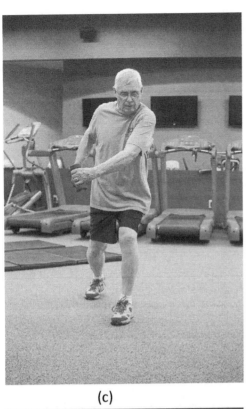

(c)

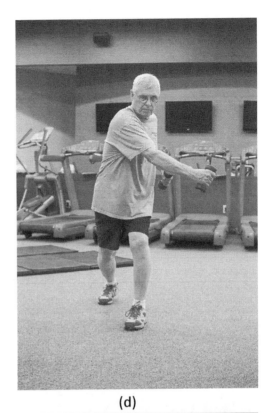

(d)

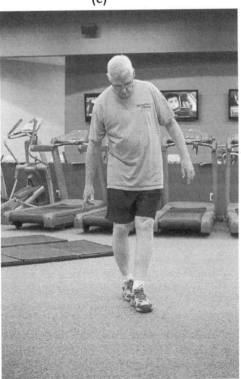

Tandem (tight-rope) walking (a)

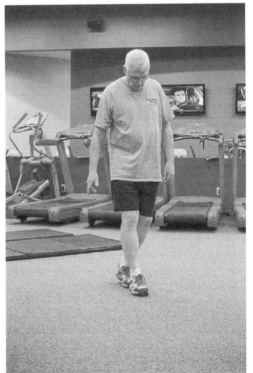

(b)

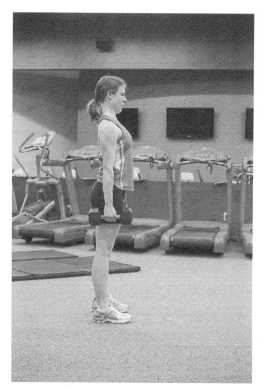 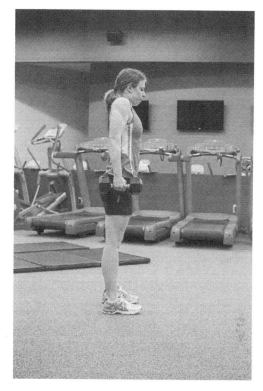

Shrugs

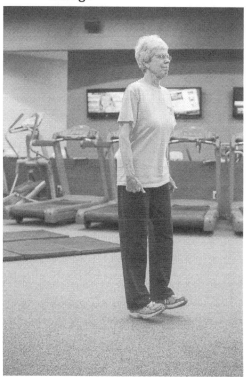 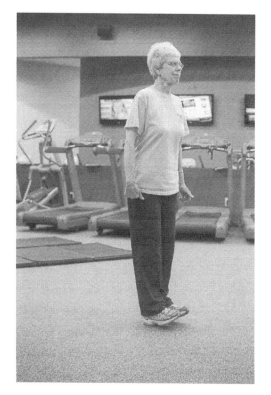

Walking on Heels

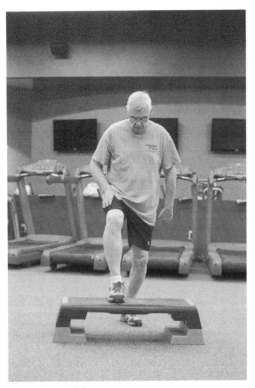

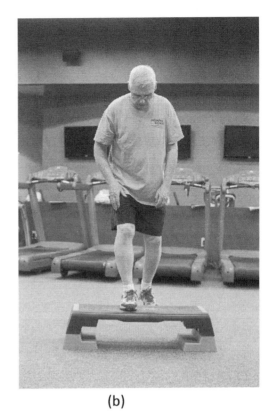

Step-Ups (a)

(b)

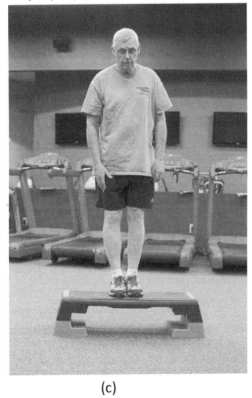

(c)

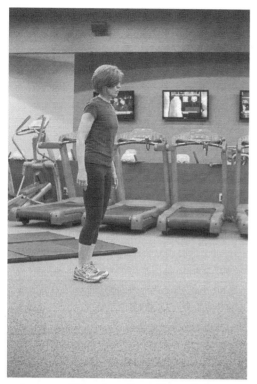

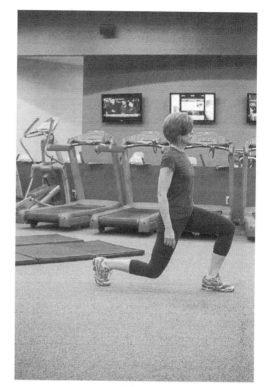

Lunges Start Small at First   (a)   (b)

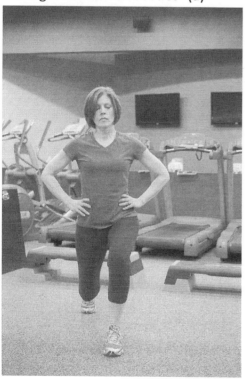

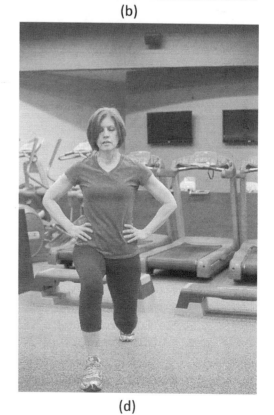

(c)   (d)

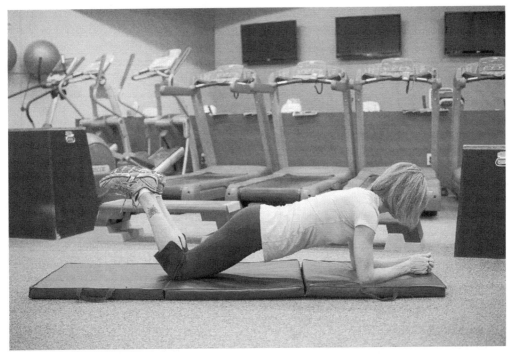

Plank On Knees   (Beginner)

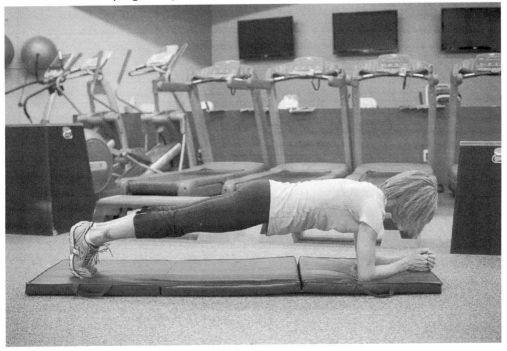

Plank on Toes (intermediate)

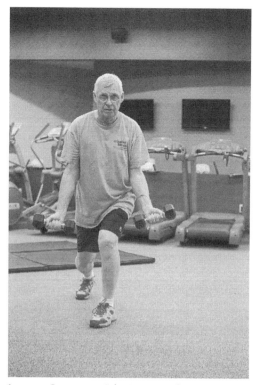
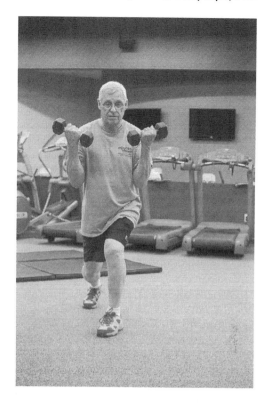

Lunge Stance with Arm Curls

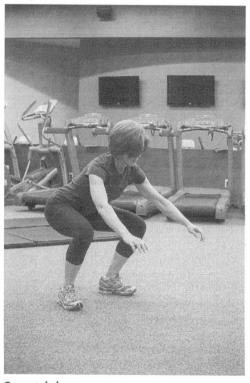
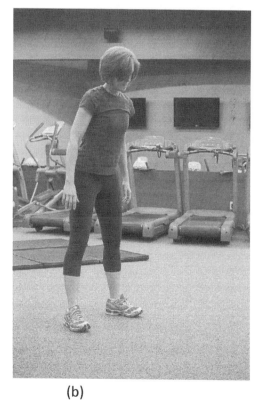

Squat (a)   (b)

Intermediate routine number 1

Stepping over a sleeping dog or parking block in all directions, forwards, backwards, sideways, diagonal

Lunges with Rotational movement

Plank: Hold your body in a plank form, on your forearms and toes

Planks with alternating leg lift and/or arm lift

Lunge stance with Arm Curl & Shoulder Press

Cable Chops: Chopping motion using a cable machine

Torso Twists using a Medball or Dumbbell

Cable Squat and Pull/Row: Using a Cable machine sit down in a squat and hold while you perform Rows/Pulls

Squats with Dumbbells

Sideways Lunges

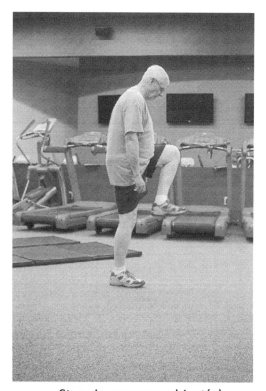

Stepping over an object(a)

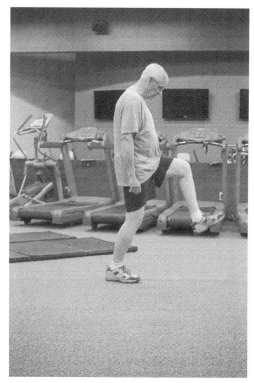

(b)

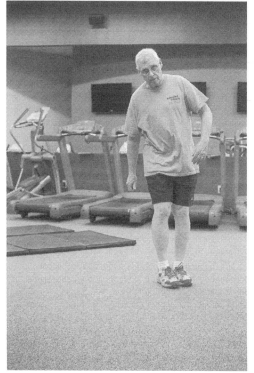

Stepping sideways (a)

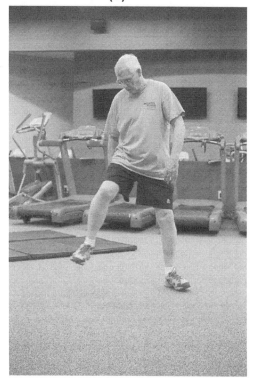

(b)

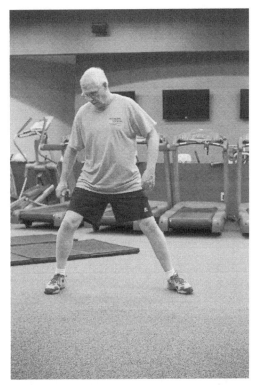

(c)

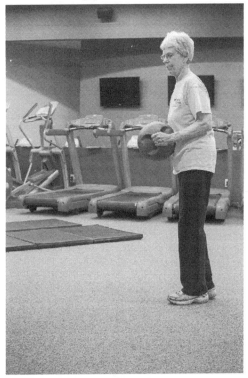

Lunges with Rotation   (a)

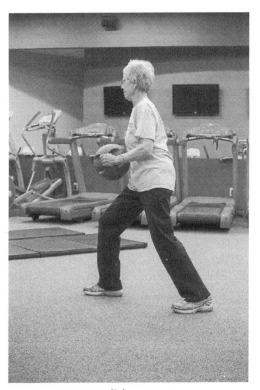

(b)

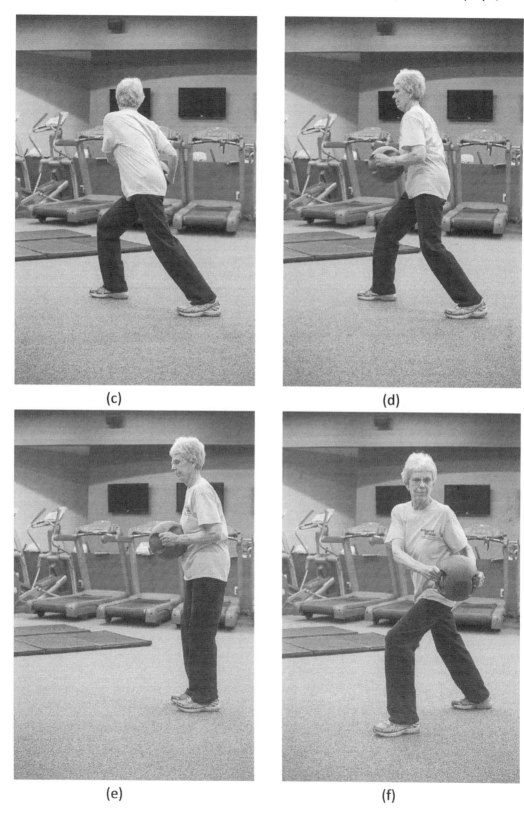

(c)

(d)

(e)

(f)

Never Grow Old!

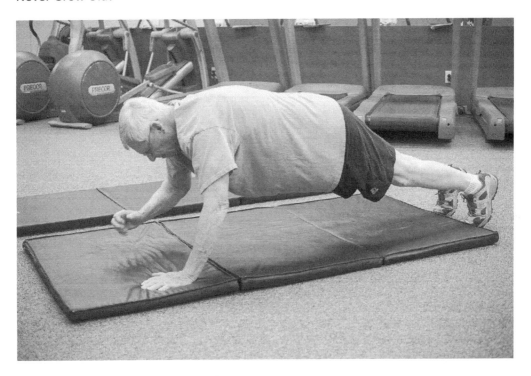

Plank Up Downs

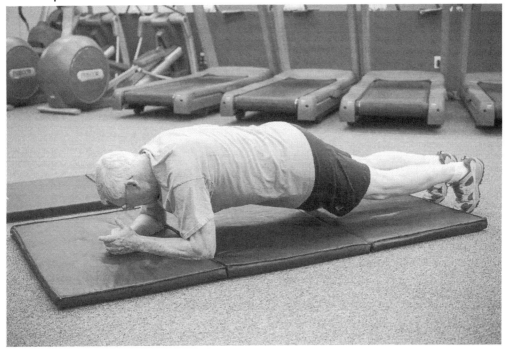

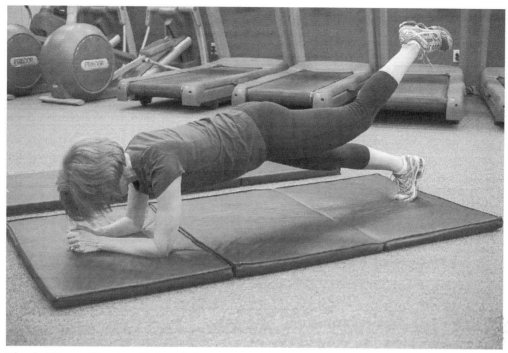

Plank Alternating Leg Raise (a)

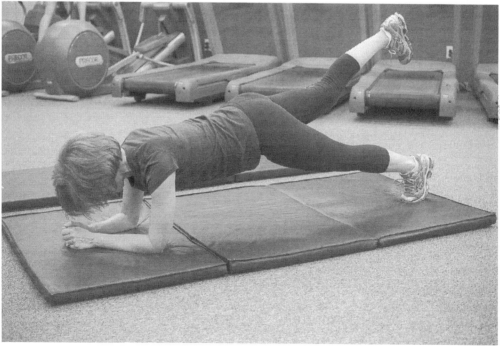

Plank Alternating Leg Raise (b)

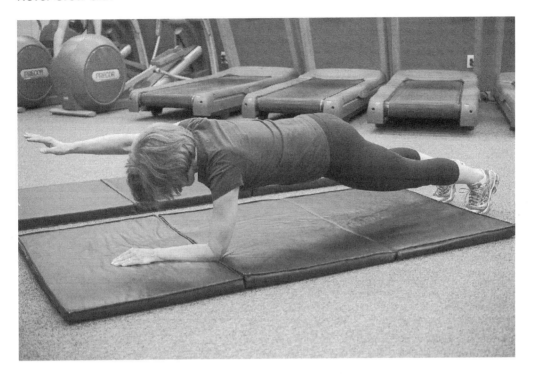

Plank alternating Arm Raise (a)

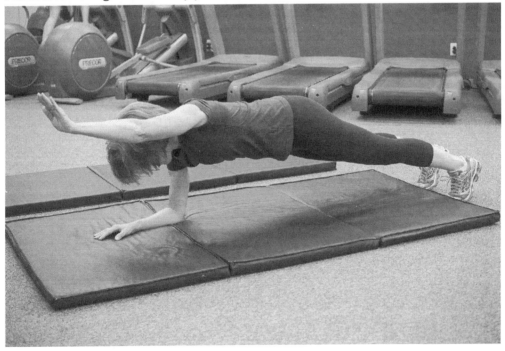

(b)

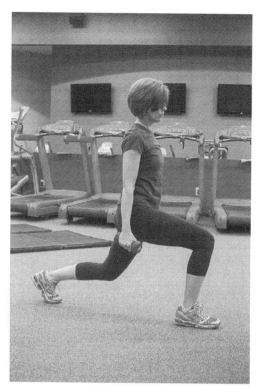
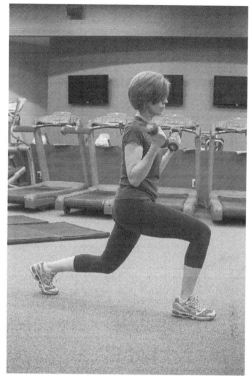

Lunge stance with arm curl and shoulder press (a)   (b)

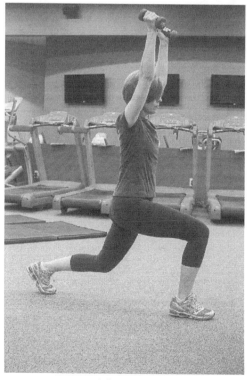
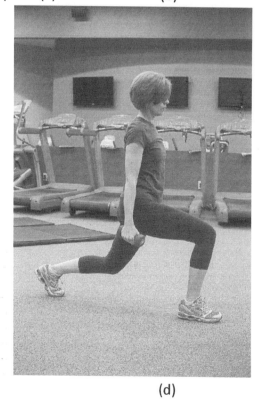

(c)   (d)

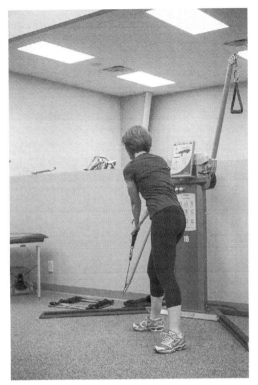

Chops (a)

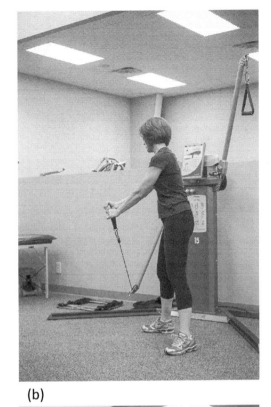

(b)

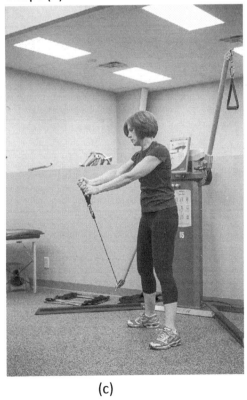

(c)

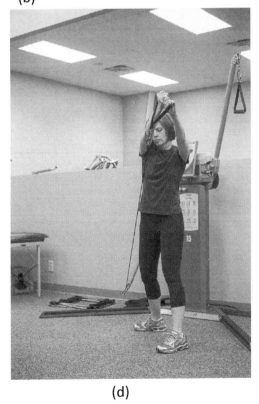

(d)

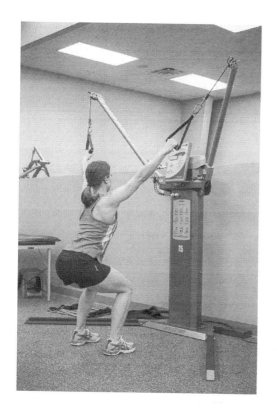 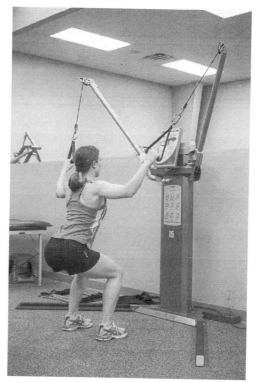

Cable Squat and Pull/Row

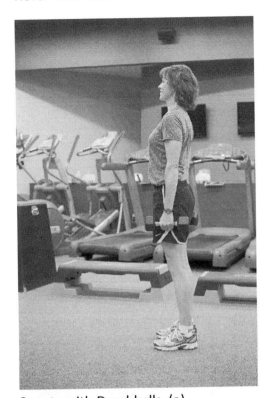

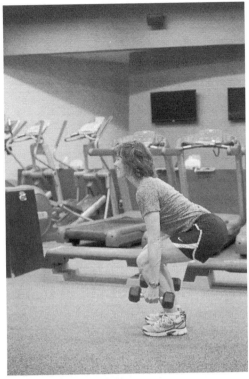

Squats with Dumbbells (a)

(b)

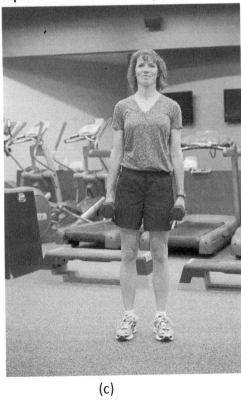

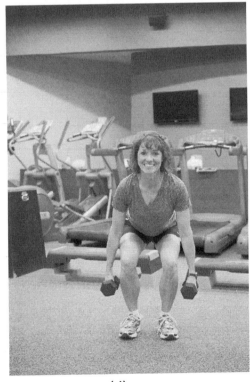

(c)

(d)

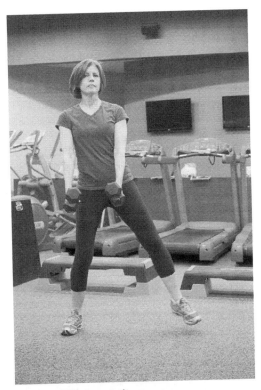

Sideways Lunges

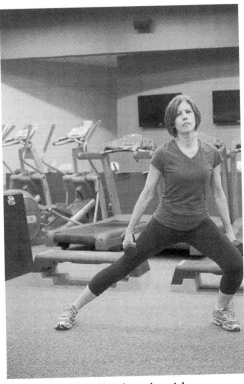

with dumbbells   hands wide

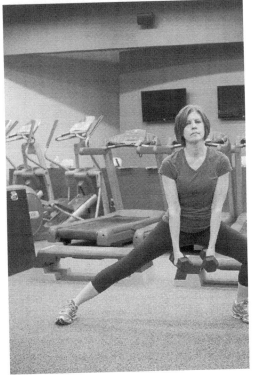

hands inside

Intermediate routine number 2

Tandem March: Similar to the Tandem Walk except now you are attempting to raise your knee up as in a march and place your feet one in front of the other.

Chair Stands with Hands Overhead

Pushups: Standard on the Toes

Rotation Twists Using a Cable

Torso Twists using a medicine ball, could use a dumbbell

Abdominal Hold: Shown using a Ball, could have hands in giant circle

Diagonal Lunges

Squat Jumps (can be done without leaving the floor, no hop)

Mountain Climbers Modified no hopping

Get Ups with no weight

Lunges with Curl and Press

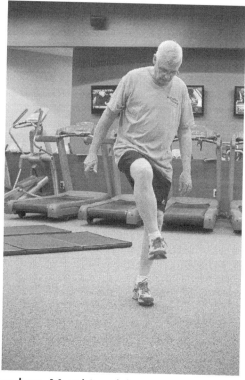 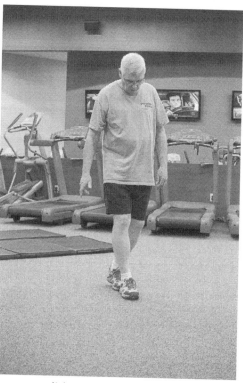

Tandem Marching (a)   (b)

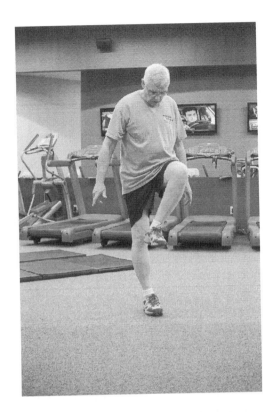
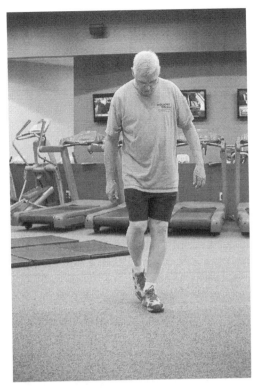

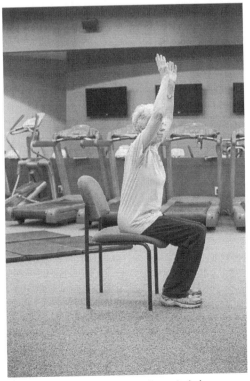
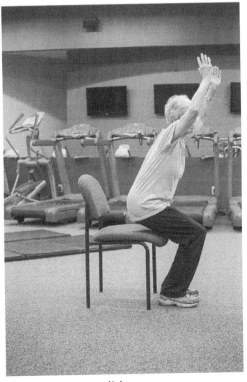

Chair Stand Arms Overhead (a)

(b)

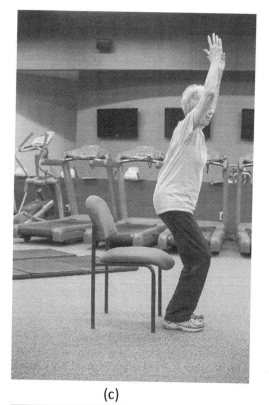

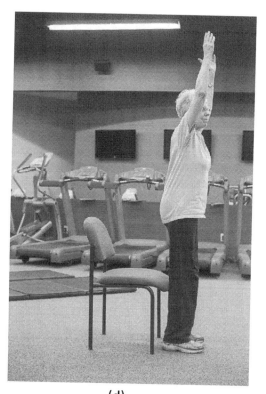

(c)

(d)

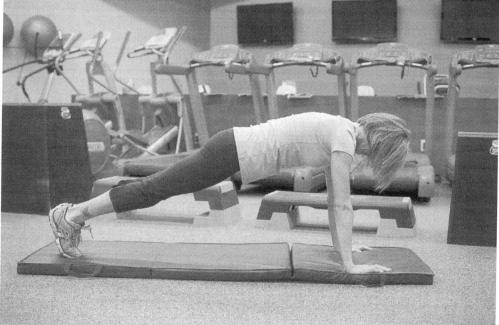

Pushups on Toes

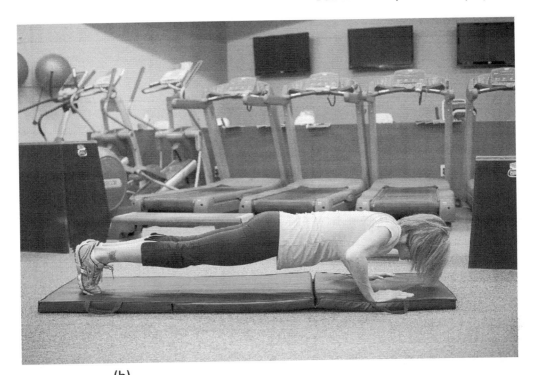

(b)

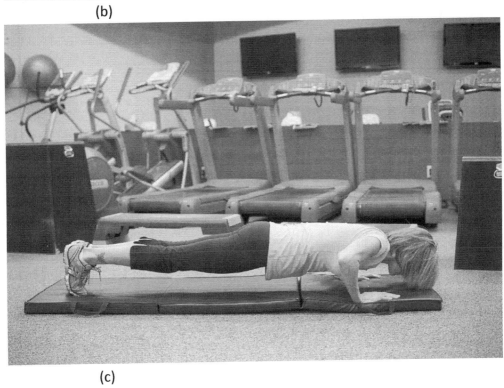

(c)

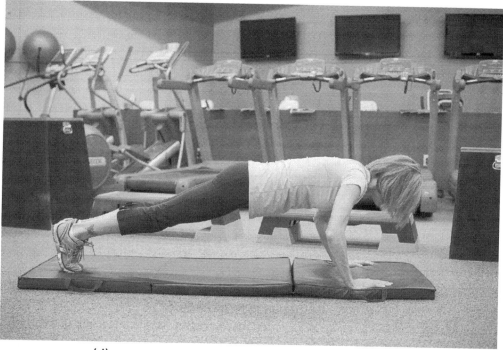

(d)

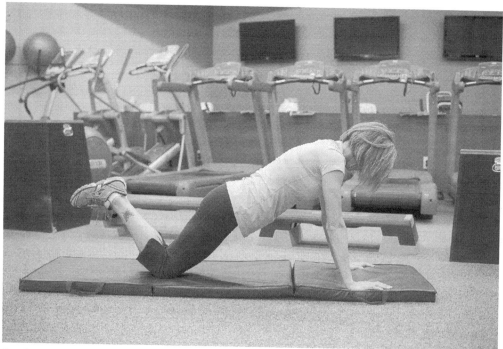

Pushups On Knees

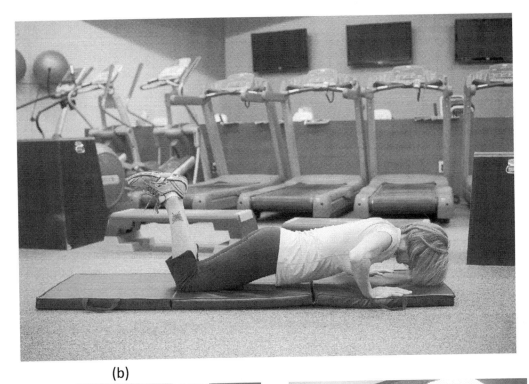

(b)

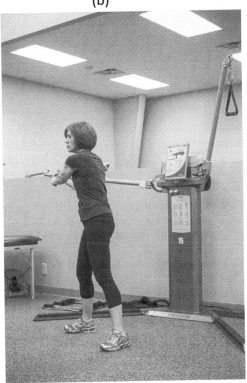

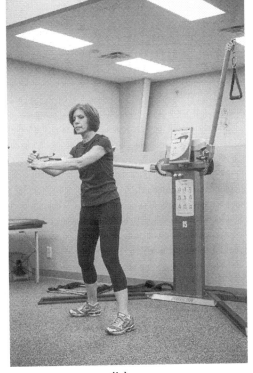

Rotational twists: Cable   (a)

(b)

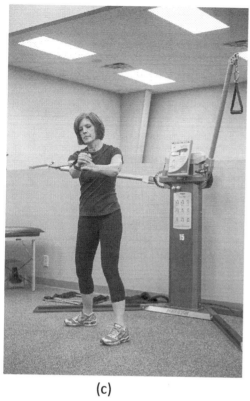

(c)

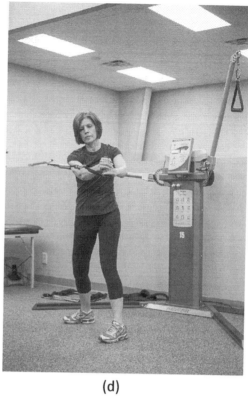

(d)

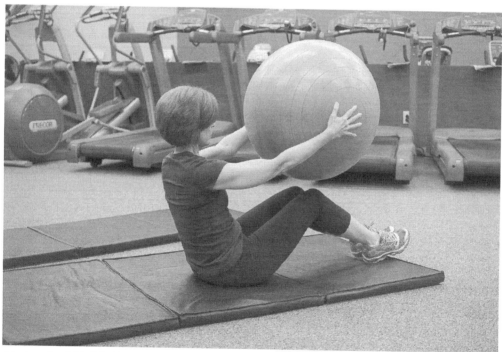

Abdominal Hold, Knees Bent Slight Lean Back Hold for Time

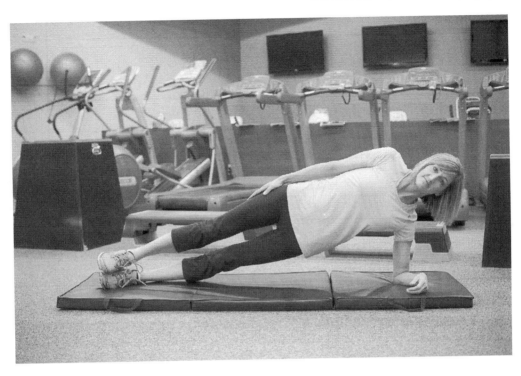

Side Plank on Feet

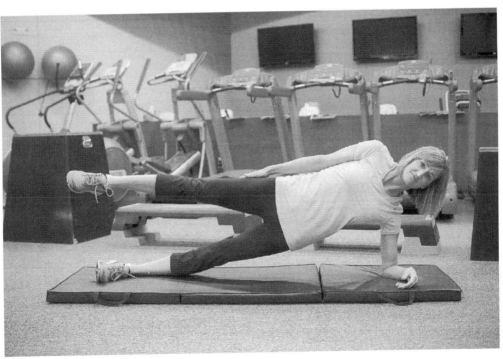

Side Plank with a Leg Lift

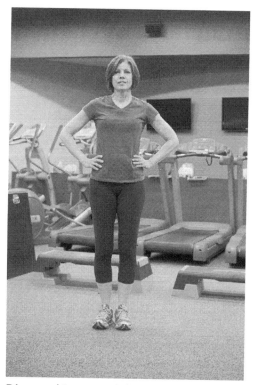

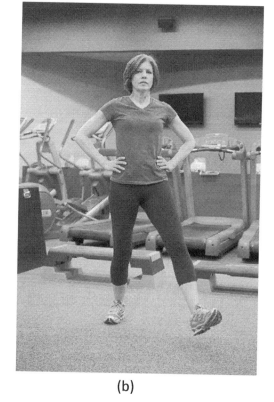

Diagonal Lunges (a)

(b)

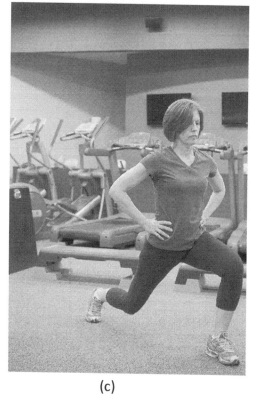

(c)

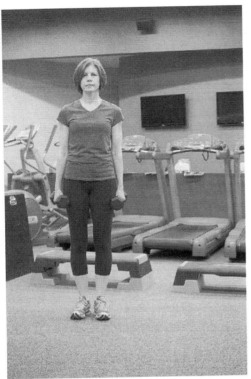

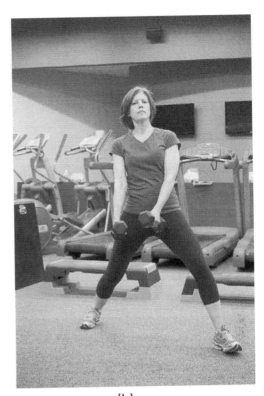

Diagonal Lunges with Dumbbells (a)

(b)

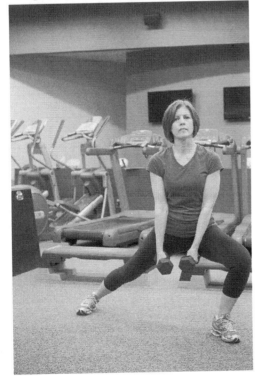

(c)

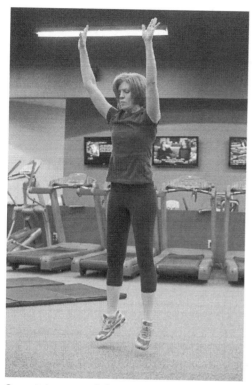
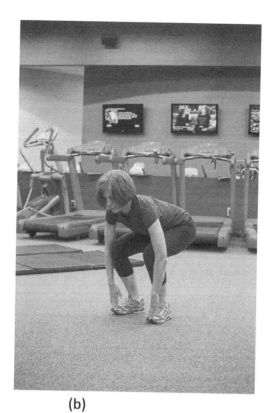

Squat Jumps   (a)   (b)

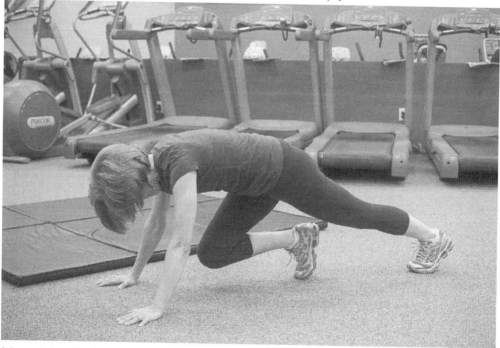

Mountain Climbers (a)

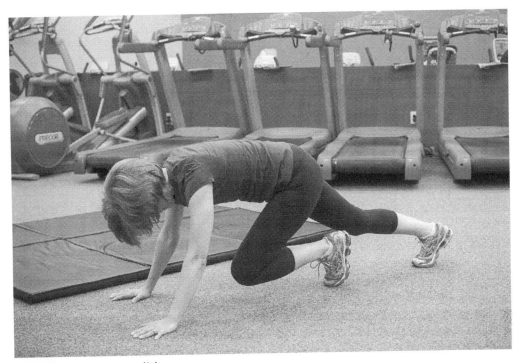

Mountain Climbers (b)

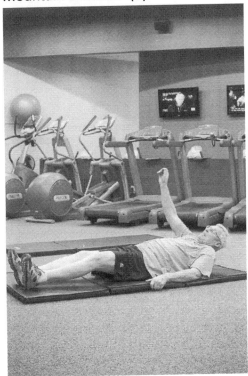

Get Ups no weight (a)

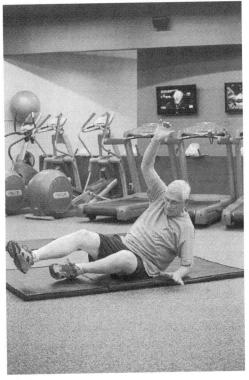

(b)

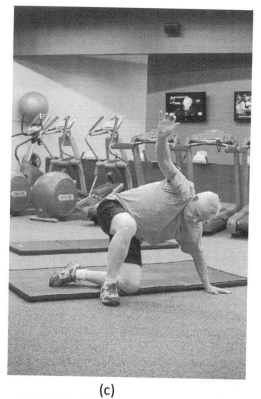

(c)

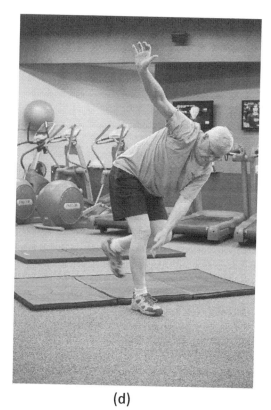

(d)

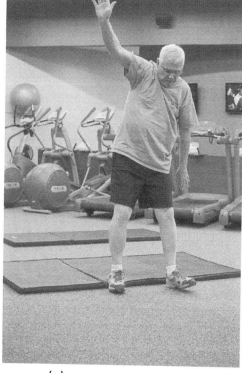

(e)

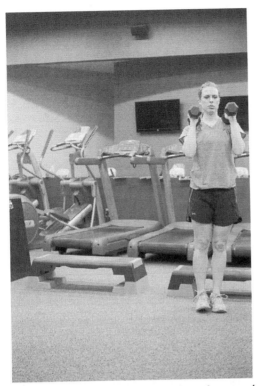

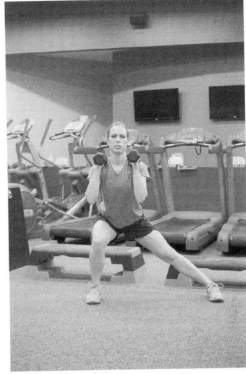

Sideways Lunges with overhead press (a)   (b)

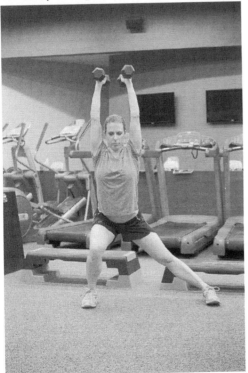

(c)

Advanced routine number 1

Plank Up Downs: Start in the Plank position and Move Up to the Standard Pushup Position, Being able to do pushups and planks well may be required to accomplish this exercise

Get Ups with Dumbbell in 1 hand: Same as Get Ups except now you have a weight to hold up toward the ceiling

Pushups: On your toes

Reverse Plank: As it sounds, this may not be comfortable for every shoulder

Kneeling One Arm Overhead Press

Modified Burgees with Dumbbells: Now you are doing the Burpee movement but you have to take dumbbells down to the floor and then back over head, no hop necessary.

Lunge with a Bent Over Row Two Arms: You can do this holding the lunch position the entire time, or performing a lunch and then a Row and repeating

One Arm Cable Punch: Standing while Pressing or Punching with one arm, use your core to steady your torso.

Burpees

Step-Ups with Overhead lift: Now you are performing step-ups while raising a weight ball over your head, we recommend you be near a wall or use a weighted object you can easily drop if necessary if you were to lose your balance you might not want to drop a dumbbell.

Mini Bench Hop/Quick Step over and back

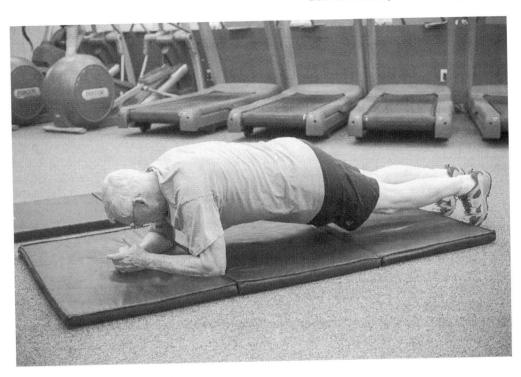

Plank Up Downs (a)

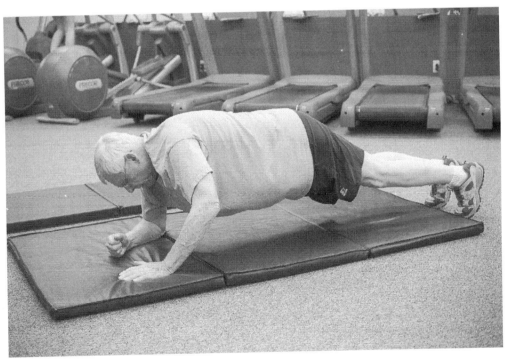

(b)

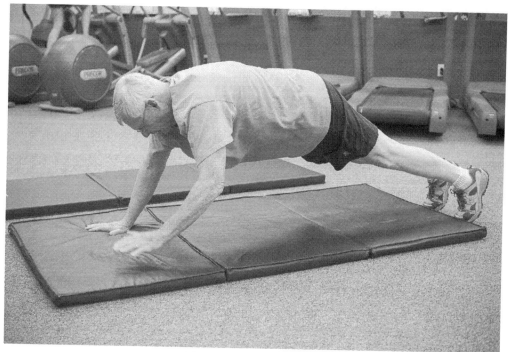

(c)

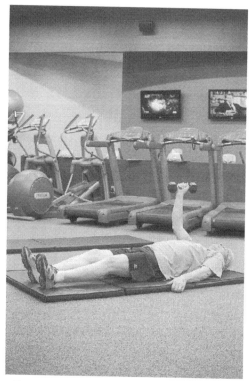

Get ups with dumbbell in 1 hand (a)

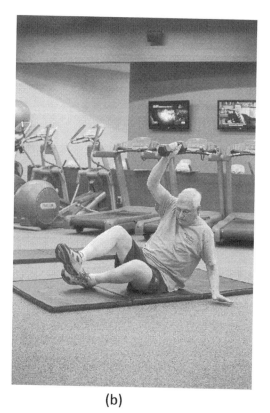

(b)

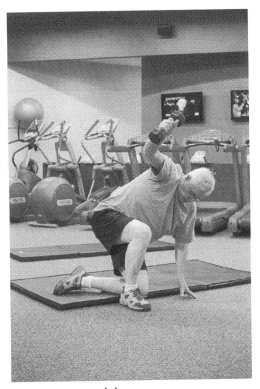

(c)

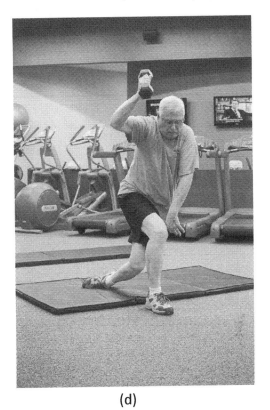

(d)

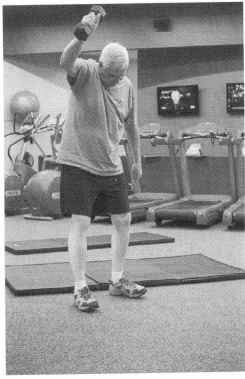

(e)

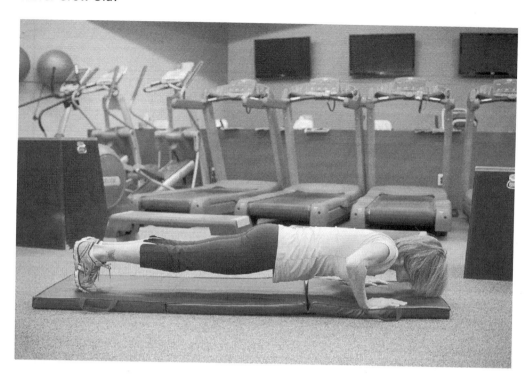

Pushups on Toes (a)

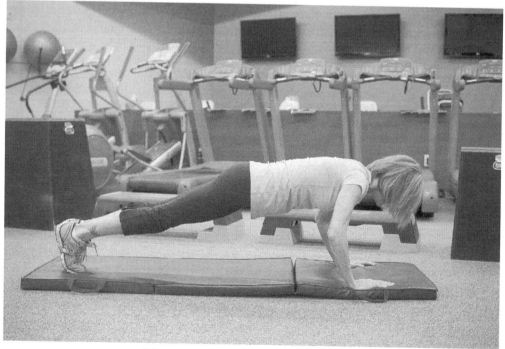

(b)

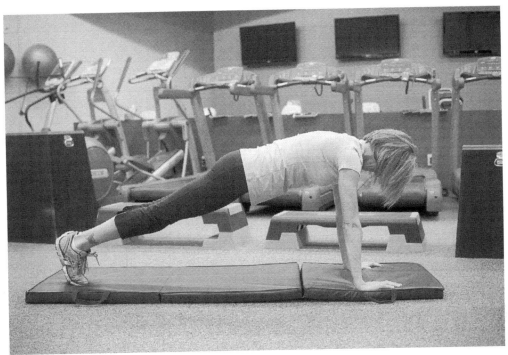

(c)

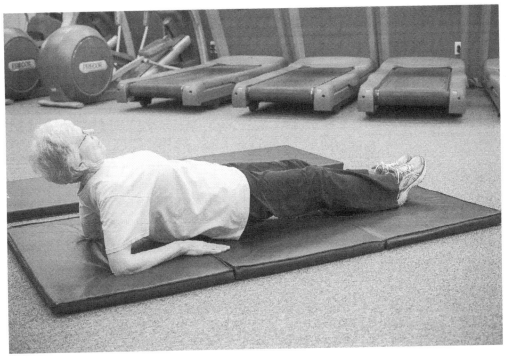

Reverse Plank

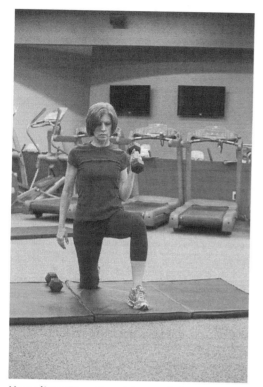
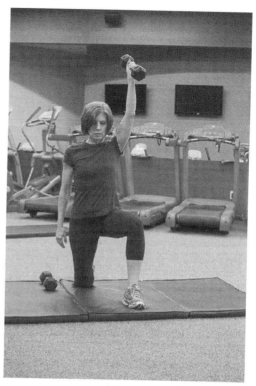

Kneeling One Arm Press (a)   (b)

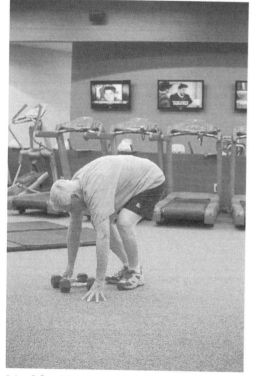
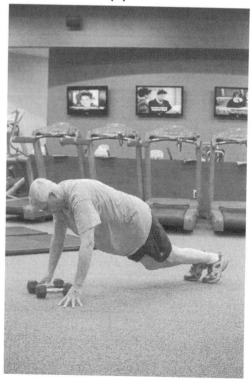

Modified Burpee with Dumbbells (a)   (b)

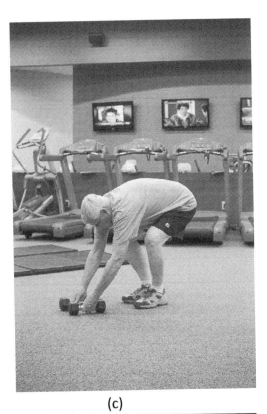

(c)

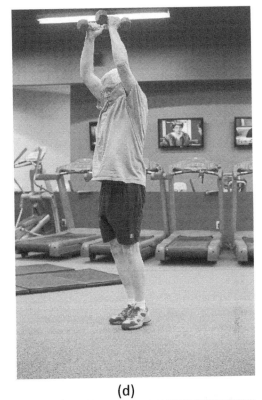

(d)

Lunge with Bent Over Row (2 Arms)

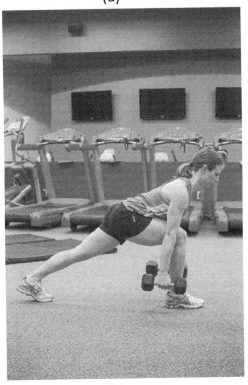

(b)

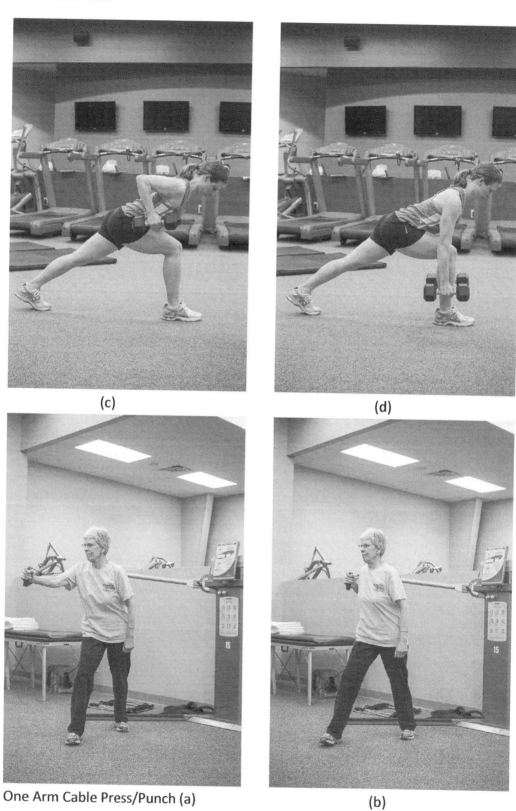

(c)

(d)

One Arm Cable Press/Punch (a)

(b)

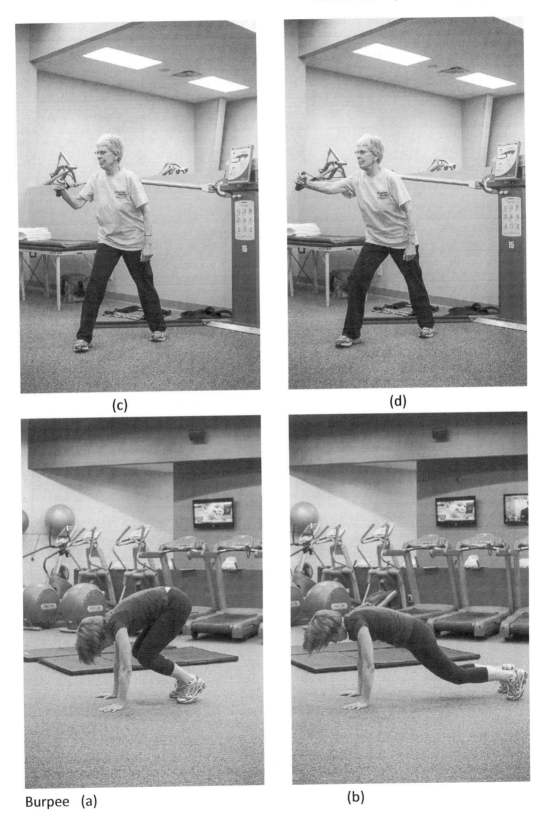

(c)

(d)

Burpee   (a)

(b)

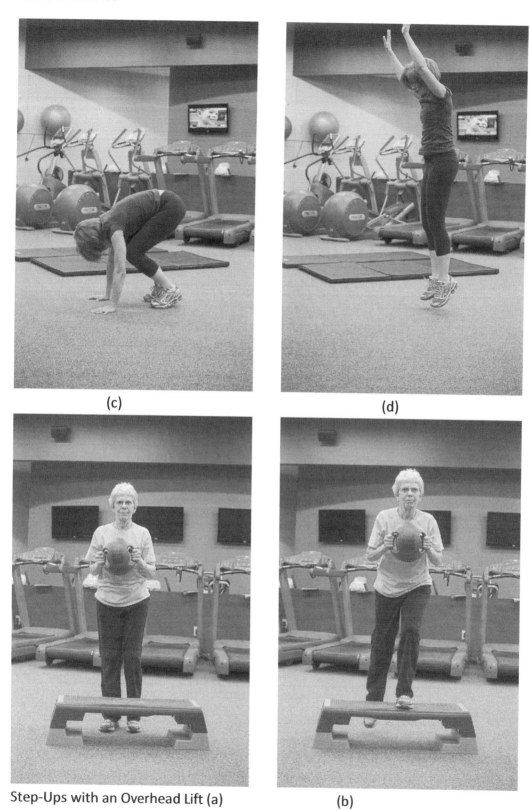

(c)

(d)

Step-Ups with an Overhead Lift (a)

(b)

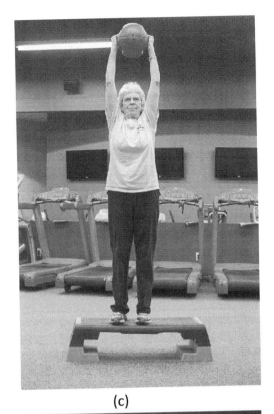

(c)

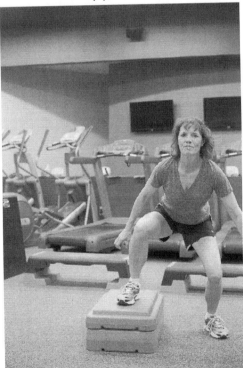

Mini Bench Hops/Steps Over and Back (a)

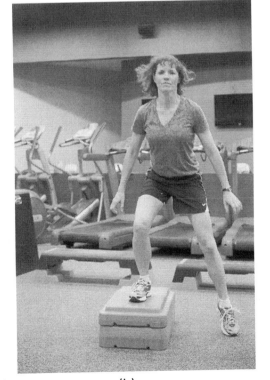

(b)

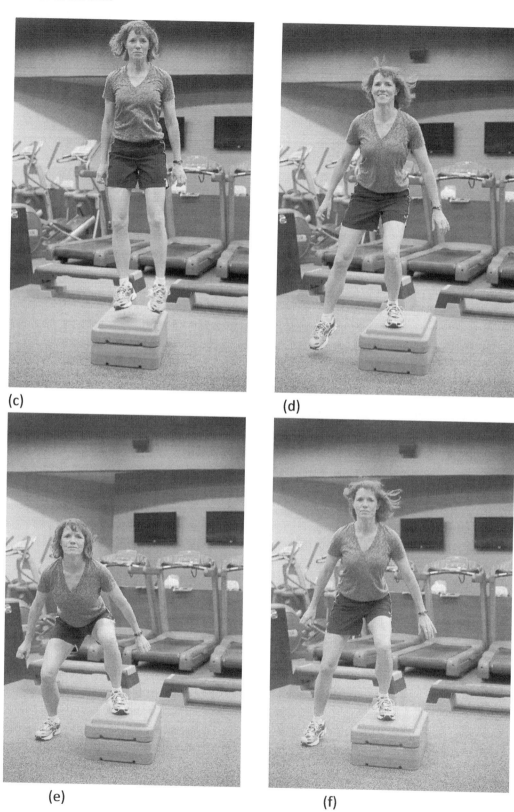

(c)

(d)

(e)

(f)

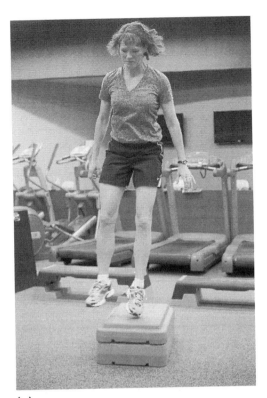

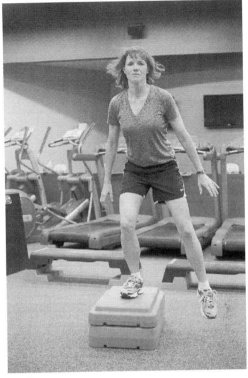

(g)

(h)

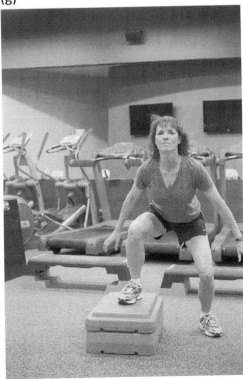

Advanced Routine number 2

Climbing Pushups: Start from the Pushup position and move one foot as close up to your hand as possible as if you are climbing a rock. Bring that foot back, and climb with your other foot, after each foot climbs perform a regular pushup then repeat.

Mountain Climbers: Start from the Pushup position and bring your foot straight forward and repeat back and forth as quick as possible as if you are running in place on the floor. When you count repetitions it is for each leg, not total, so perform 15 for each leg.

Burpees

Lunges

Leg Curl with Ball: Lying on your back lift your hips up into the bridge position with your feet on the ball now. Once in the bridge position bring the ball in towards you bending your knees. At first have your hands spread wide for a nice stable base of support. To make it progressively more challenging bring your hands in closer to your body and eventually take your hands off the mat.

Straight Leg Lift with Ball: Again lying on your back lift your hips up into a bridge position, then keep your legs straight slowing lift your legs about 1-2 feet off the ball, alternating. Hint the leg staying on the ball will work harder than the leg you are lifting.

Side Plank: Perform a Plank on your side on just one arm

Torso Twist with your feet up in the air

Sideways Lunge Reach and Crossover and finish with a Knee Raise: This is a complicated movement lunge sideways and then reach across your foot outside and then follow through ending with a knee raise.

Cable Chest Press two arms while standing in a Lunge Stance: Holding a lunge stance Press both cable out in front of you, be sure to use your core to maintain your posture.

Pulldown with a Split Stance

Step-Up With Overhead Lift: Now you are performing step-ups while raising a weighted ball over your head, we recommend you be near a wall or use a weighted object you can easily discard, if you lose your balance you don't want to have to drop a dumbbell.

Lunge with an overhead press, shown from various angles. Again to make more challenging perform each lunge for every overhead press repetition.

Reverse crossover punch: maintain a shoulder width stand while reach/cross over behind you with a dumbbell.

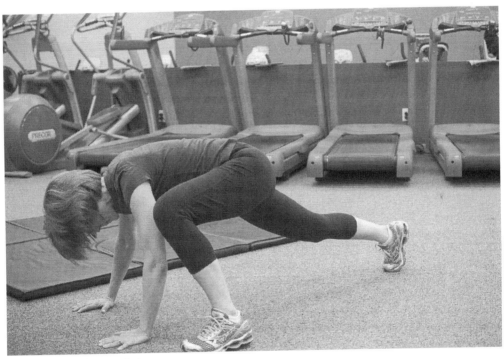

Climbing Push-ups (a)

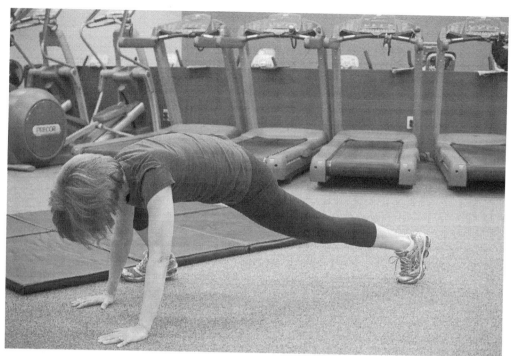

(b)

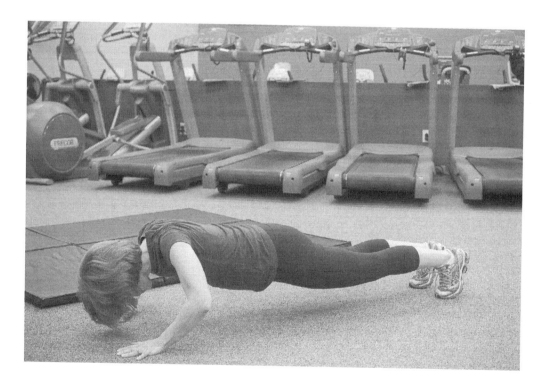

(c)

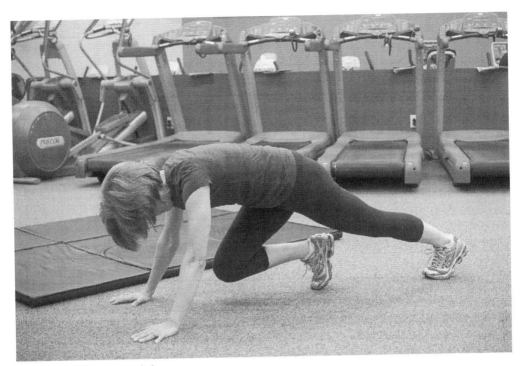

Mountain Climbers (a)

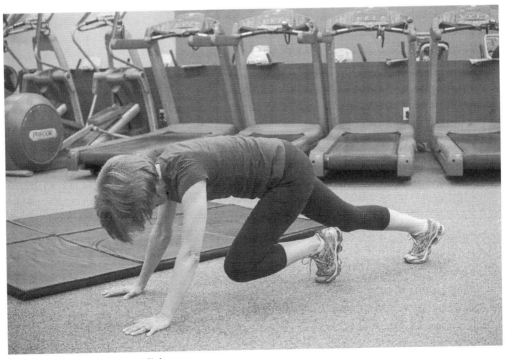

(b)

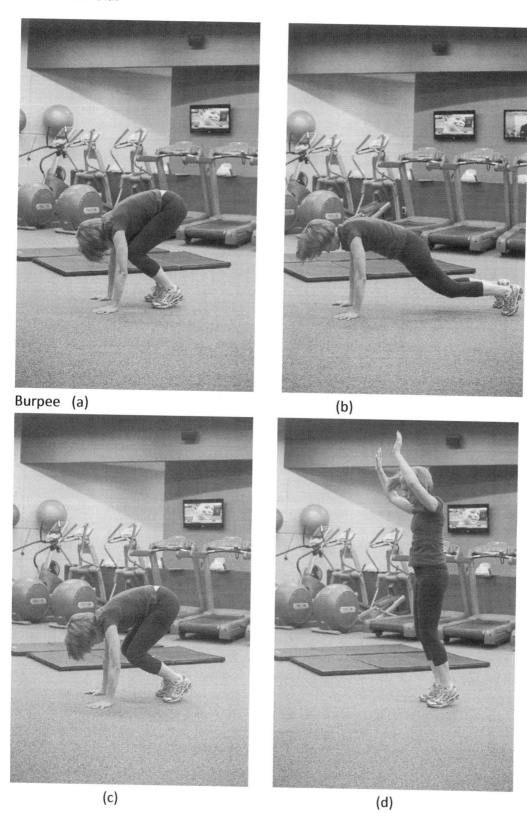

Burpee (a)

(b)

(c)

(d)

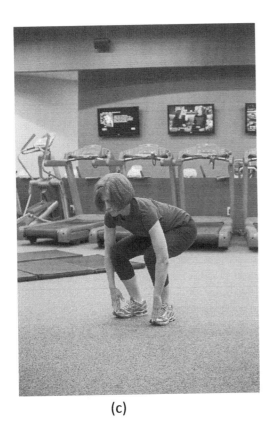

(c)

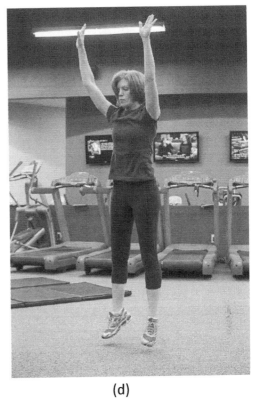

(d)

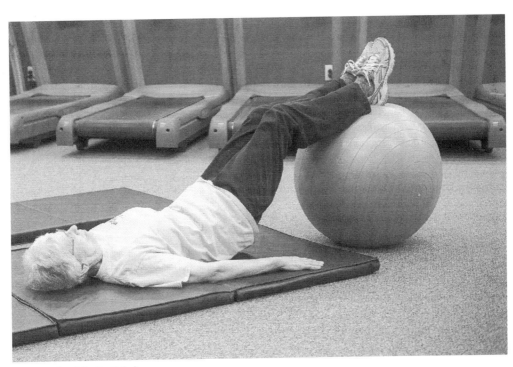

Leg curl with Ball (a)

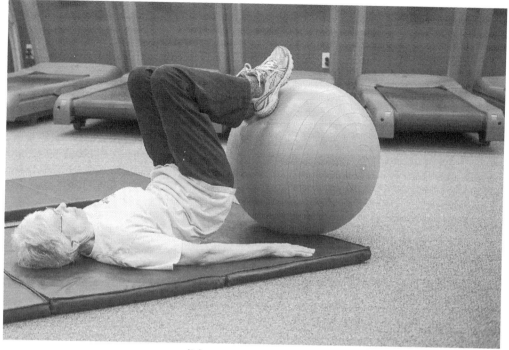

(b)

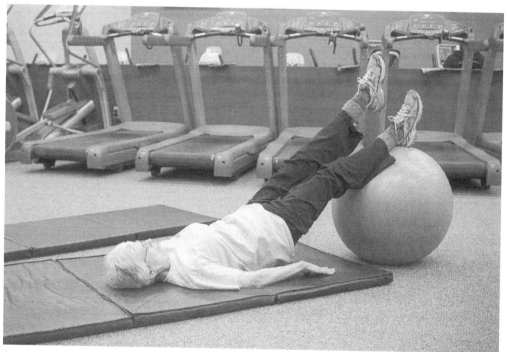

Straight Leg Lift w Ball (a)

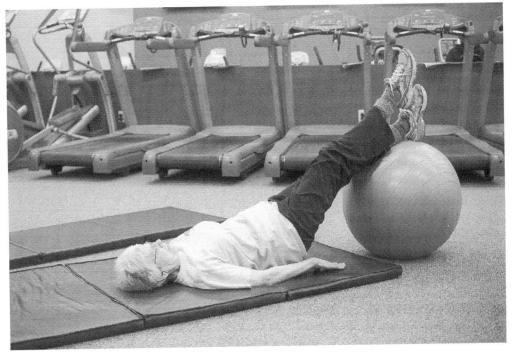

(b)

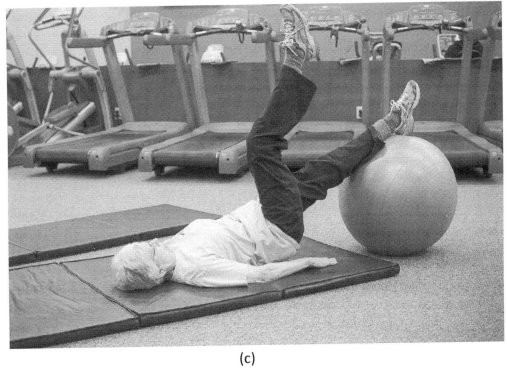

(c)

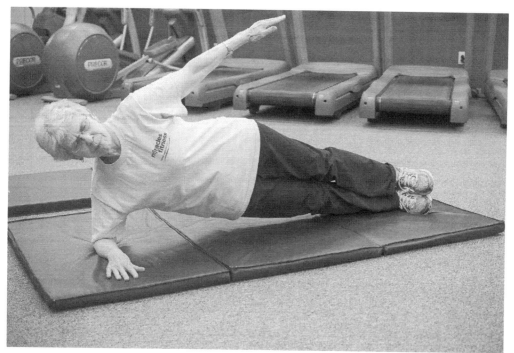

SidePlank

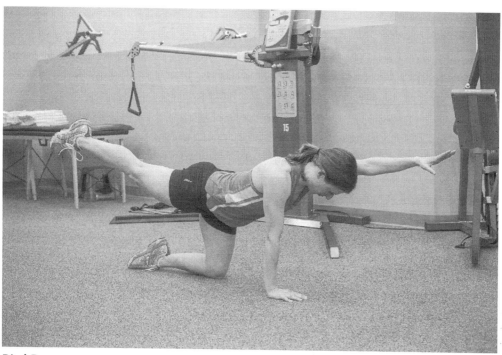

Bird Dog

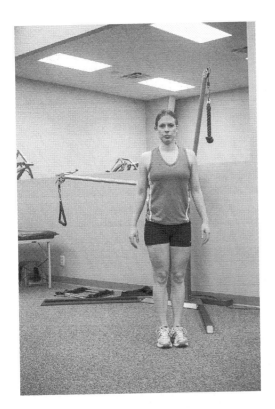
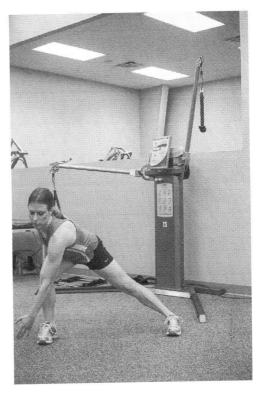
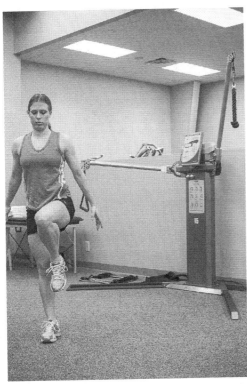

Sideways Lunge with a Crossover Reach Finishing with a Knee Raise

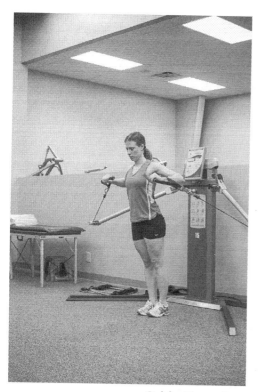 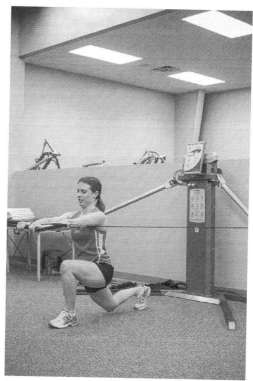

Cable Chest Press with a Lunge

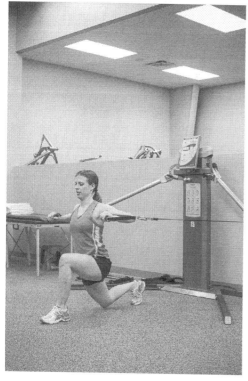

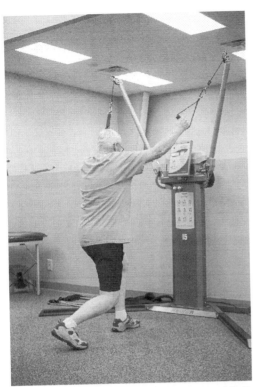
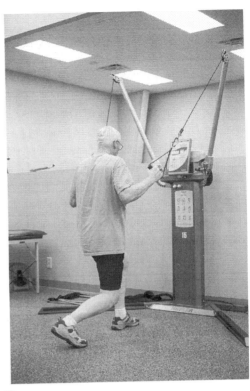

Pulldown with Split Stance

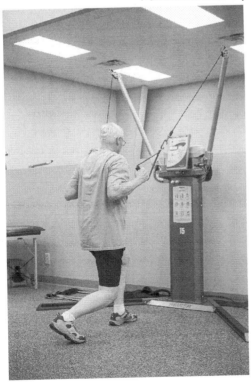

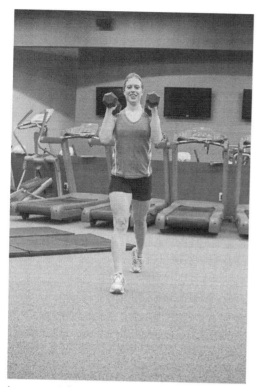

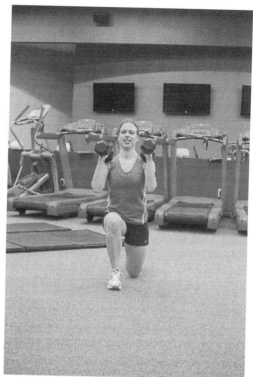

Lunge with Overhead Press Hands in Close   (b)

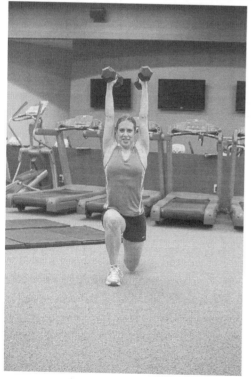

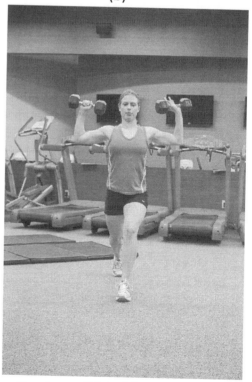

c)   Hands out Wide (a)

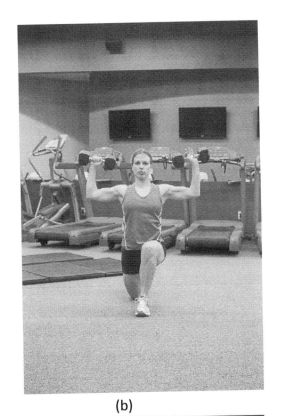

(b)

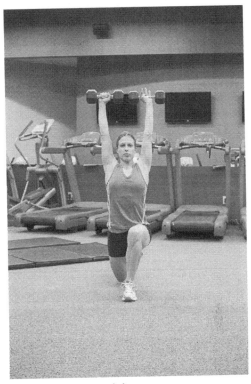

(c)

Hands Wide Side View   (a)

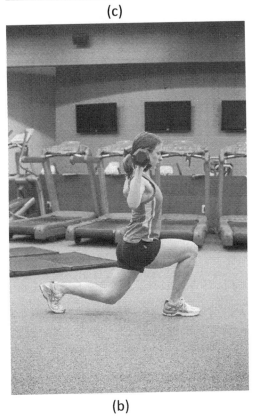

(b)

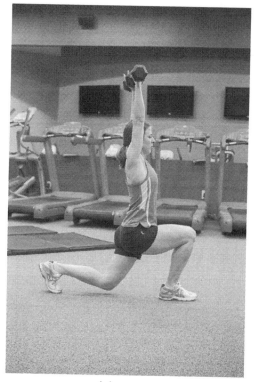

(c)

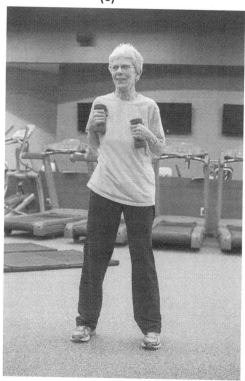

Reverse Crossover Punch (a)

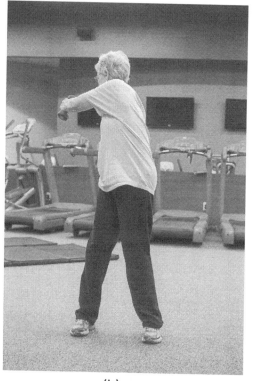

(b)

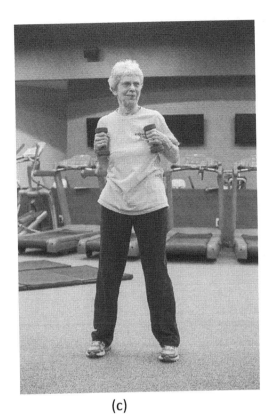

(c)

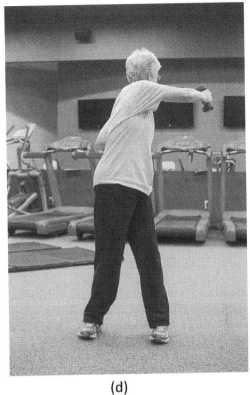

(d)

Bonus Exercises

We included a few more exercises just for substitution.

Some of these you may need to substitute if you find certain exercises too hard, or if you have trouble lifting things over your head due to shoulder problems.

Some are just variations of exercises we have already shown.

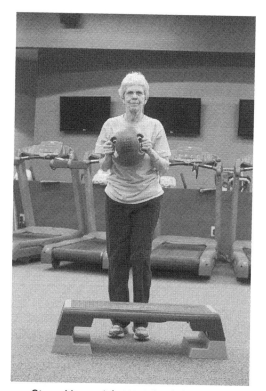

Step-Ups with Weight (a)

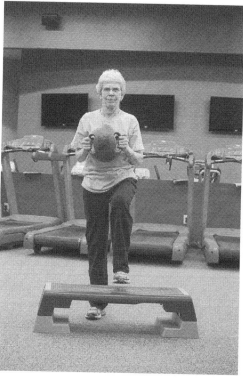

(b)

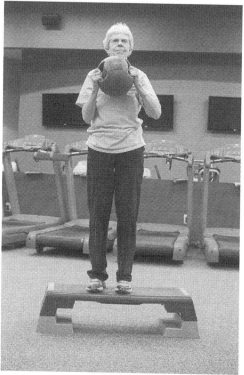

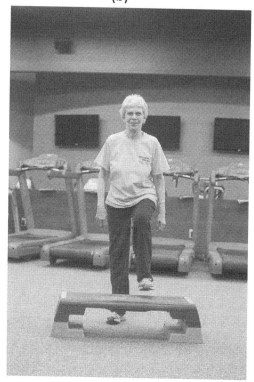

Step Up with Knee Raise (a)

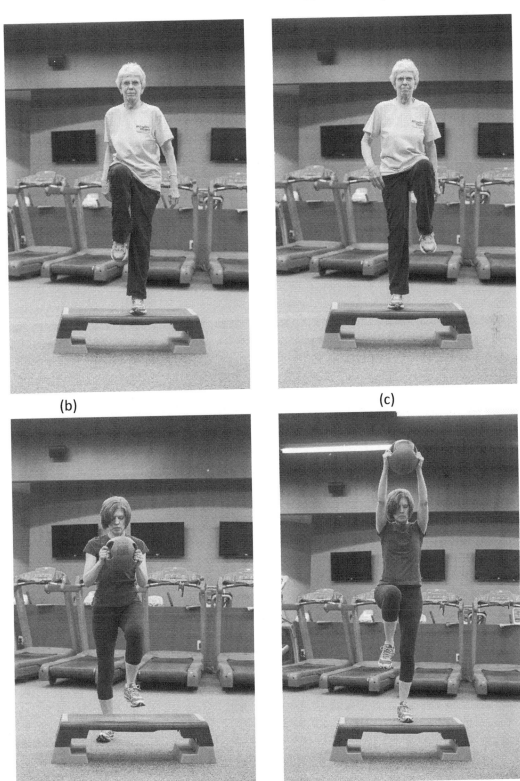

(b)   (c)

Step-Ups With OverHead Lift and Knee Raise

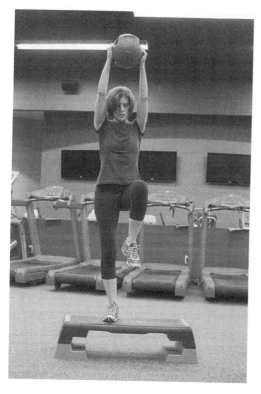

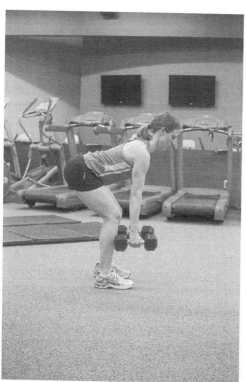
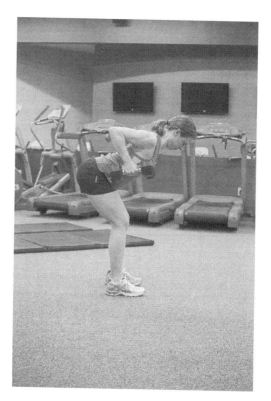

Bent Over Rows Two Arms

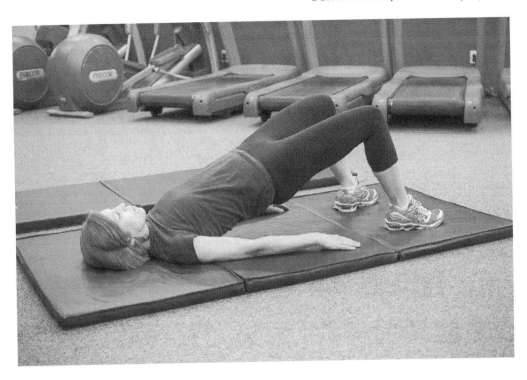

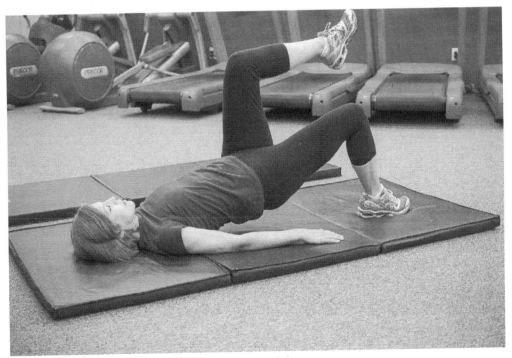

Bridge with alternating March/Knee Raise (a)

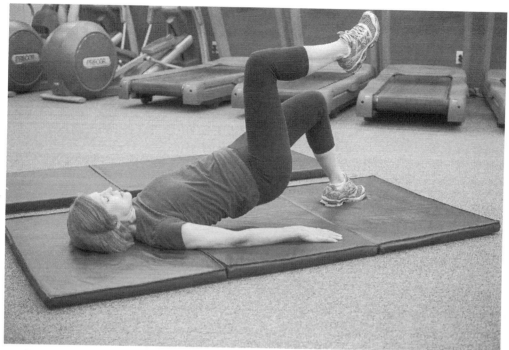

Bridge with alternating March/Knee Raise (b)

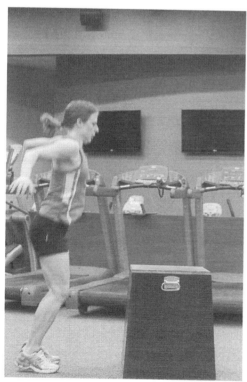

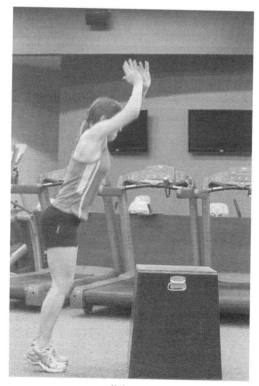

Box Jump Take Off   (a)   (b)

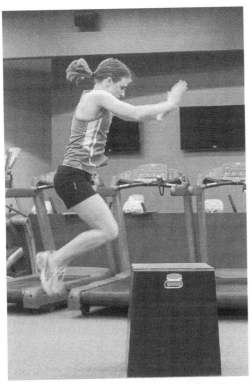

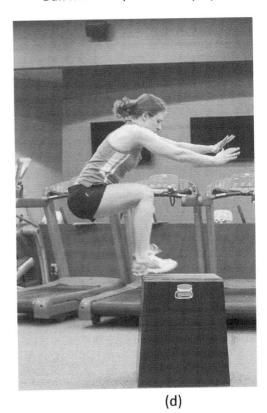

(c)   Box jump   (d)

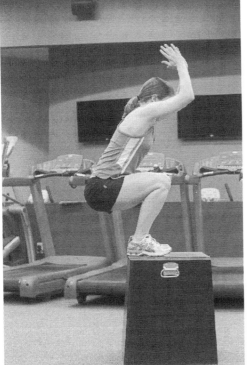

Landing (e)

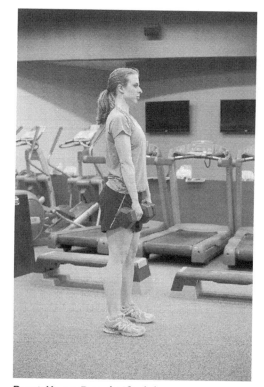
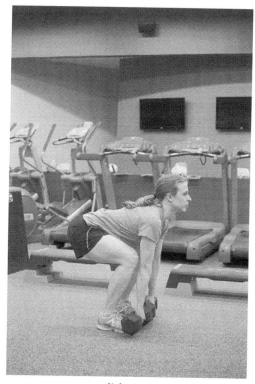

Bent Knee Dead Lift (a)   (b)

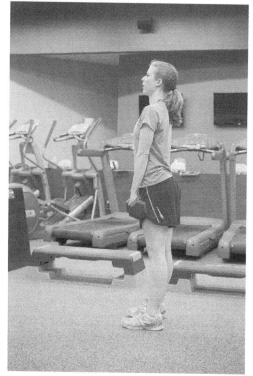
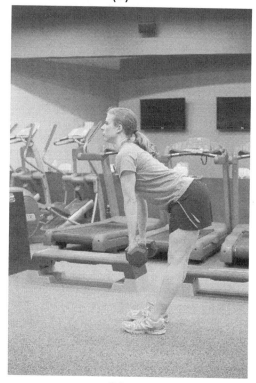

Straight Leg Dead Lift   (a)   (b)

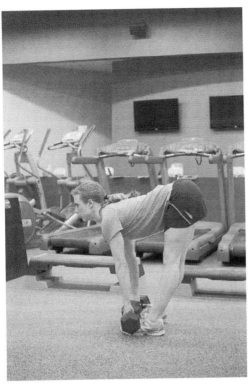

(c)

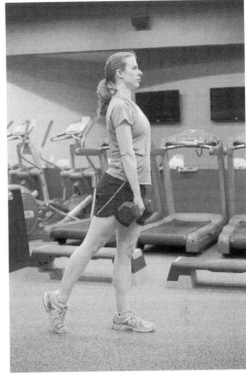

Single Leg Stiff Leg Dead Lift (a)

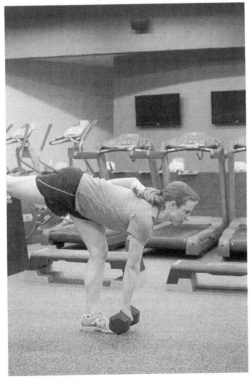

(b)

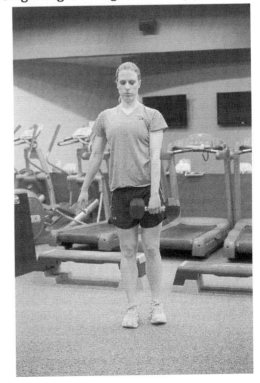

Never Grow Old!

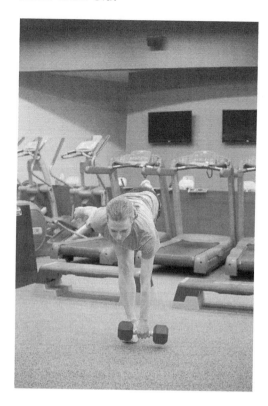

Okay so now we have given you several exercise routines, lets recap and review. First keep in mind your safety is our utmost concern, this book is of no use to you if you wind up hurting yourself. So please keep in mind some exercises shown may not be appropriate for you maybe because of shoulder issues, or knee pain. Please do not take the "I'll tough it out approach". Remember chapter 2 Principle #7 Be safe to be successful.

Now lets think about the Principles in action. Principle #2 : Make purposeful decisions for every aspect of training. So lets talk briefly about what that might mean for you. If you want to be able to get down on the floor and spend more time with your grandchildren some exercises related to getting on the floor, being on the floor and getting up from the floor will have more importance for you. If you want to swing a golf club with less back pain and be able to hit the ball farther more standing exercises with rotational (twisting) movements will be important for you. If you are having trouble with balance or have even fallen recently then spending more focused time on balance specific exercises may be of most importance for you.

This doesn't mean you do only the exercises specific to your main goals, but it does mean you might choose to do more sets of those or begin to add more of those exercises into your routines. Again like we stated in the beginning on this chapter we expect that you will use a proper warm-up before beginning any of these exercise routines. We included one for you, but you may already have a warm-up routine you prefer. As you get more advanced you may want to use some of the beginner workouts as your warm-up exercises. We would encourage you to begin with the beginner routines and progress to the intermediate as soon as you feel you are easily mastering the beginner routines and similarly on to the advanced routines. If you would prefer to have some fitness tests we encourage you to see our Resources page at the back of the book. It is always important to be changing your exercise routine. You do not want to do the same exercise routine over and over and over. I would encourage you to mix in another exercise every time and switch from one routine to another. We would not expect it to take months to progress from the beginner to intermediate routines. Keep in mind there are several ways you can make your exercise progressively harder. Add more resistance if you started out doing an exercise with no resistance you can add a dumbbell or medicine ball to give more resistance. If you are using resistance presently simply increasing the resistance accordingly. In addition you can increase the number of repetitions and also add a 2nd or 3rd set of the same exercise. Additionally use our resource page for many new exercise routines and visual displays of more exercises. We have only included 2 routines at each level, as a starting point, so please visit our website often for more and more exercise routines.

Do not pick a routine and do that over and over and over again for months. For maximal results you need variety and progressions. It is as simple to say if you don't have a plan to progress, you aren't likely to make much progress. For more workout routines in video format please visit our website: www.functionalfitnesssolution.com.

Chapter 5: No More Slow (boring) Cardio

"Run, Forrest, Run!". You might remember this famous line from the hit movie Forrest Gump starring Tom Hanks as Forrest and Sally Field as his mother. I can vividly recall Tom Hanks running down that country lane in slow motion as his leg braces fall to pieces.   (By the way, did you know that Sally was only 10 years older than Tom when she played his mother in that movie) From that moment on Forrest became a running fool. He ran almost everywhere just because he could and because he apparently liked to.

I am no Forrest Gump that's for sure. I don't like running (it hurts my knees and hips) and I'm not too excited about any kind of cardio exercise in general. Like many of my clients I used to dread doing my cardio routine. It was long and boring. So, a number of years ago I started looking for a better option and that's when I came across some research on high-intensity interval training (HIIT).

The benefits were pretty impressive compared to the usual 30-40 minutes plodding along on the treadmill including:

- Larger and faster improvements in cardiovascular fitness
- More calories burned in a shorter period of time
- Greater amounts of body fat loss
- Greater improvements in metabolism

I tried out a few different HIIT programs and believe it or not I really liked it. So I tried out more programs and ended up getting great results. Being the academic type, I continued to search the literature to learn all I could about interval training and began to speak at fitness conferences to teach other trainers how to use them with their clients. Simultaneously I started using it with my clients. They liked it and got great results just as I had. When we opened Miracles Fitness we made HIIT a critical part of our fitness philosophy. Since then we have used it successfully with hundreds of clients of all ages, fitness levels and abilities. Many of whom (like myself) hated cardio before trying HIIT.

Other benefits that I've gleaned from my years of experience with HIIT include:

- Workouts seem to fly by rather than drag on
- I don't need to read or watch TV in order to distract me from my routine…just a little motivating music is all I need
- I feel more in tune with my body
- I look forward to cardio days instead of dreading them
- Since the workouts are shorter I spend less time at the gym and more time with family

So exactly what is HIIT?

High Intensity Interval Training

This form of interval training simply involves periods of higher-intensity exercise (exercise intervals) alternated with periods of lower-intensity exercise (recovery periods) within the same exercise session. How challenging and how long these periods last vary depending on the person's goals and abilities. Typically they are prescribed as a ratio such as 3:1 (e.g. 3 minutes of higher-intensity followed by 1 minute of recovery) or 2:1 (e.g. 60 seconds of higher-intensity followed by 30 seconds of recovery). The more intense the exercise is the shorter it needs to be (because you cannot sustain intense exercise for very long) and the longer the rest period (in comparison to the exercise interval period) needs to be. Think about it this way. An all-out sprint of 100 yards would take the average individual about 15 seconds. But they would get so out of breath that they would need to rest for about 2-3 minutes or longer before they would be ready for the next sprint. That would be a ratio of 1:8 – 1:12.

Conversely, if you just jogged the same distance and took 30 seconds to do so you might only need a minute before you were ready to jog again because you wouldn't get out of breath nearly as much. That would be a ratio of only 1:2.

How does it work?

During the exercise intervals (periods of high intensity exercise) heart rate and metabolism increase significantly. However, this level of exertion is difficult to maintain because the person gets out of breath. During the periods of recovery (lower-intensity exercise) heart rate, oxygen usage and metabolism remain elevated above the level that you would expect from the low-intensity exercise. Imagine if you had to run (or walk briskly) a couple blocks in order to catch up to a friend. Once you got there you would be breathing hard with your heart pounding fast in your chest and it would take several minutes of rest before they recovered to normal levels. Even though you are standing still, you are burning way more calories compared to what you were burning while standing still before the little run. We call this extra calorie usage "the afterburn".

Here is a principle you need to remember: The greater the intensity during the workout the greater the afterburn. It is kind of like shaking a snow globe. If you give it just a little shake then you don't disturb all of the flakes and the snow disappears quickly. But, if you give it a vigorous shake you disturb many more flakes and with the water swirling violently around inside it takes much longer for the snow to disappear. Exercise "shakes up" your metabolism and the harder you exercise the more calories you burn afterwards.

In addition, the afterburn specifically targets fat calories due to a neat phenomenon called the crossover effect. During high-intensity aerobic exercise you use more calories, as a percentage, from carbohydrates than from fat in the body. During lower-intensity exercise you use more calories, as a percentage, from fat than from carbohydrates in the body. It is easy to be misled in thinking then that lower-intensity exercise would be better for fat loss because more fat is used as energy. However, that is false for two reasons. The first reason is that although you use a lower percentage of calories from fat during higher-intensity exercise you are burning calories much faster so this partially offsets the change in percentage. Secondly, because of the after-burn, following high-intensity aerobic exercise that uses lots of carbohydrates your body decides to save as much carbohydrate as it can and switches (or crosses over) to using fat as an energy source. Since the afterburn has been shown to last for 24 hours or more, you end up burning a lot more fat AFTER the exercise session than you did DURING the exercise session. The crossover effect combined with the after-burn is a very powerful 1-2 punch for losing body fat.

HIIT Program Basics

Gauging intensity is pretty important for HIIT to be successful. Exercise too easy and you will not reap all of the benefits of the method. Exercise too hard and you won't be able to recover enough to complete the entire routine. I like to use Rating of Perceived of Exertion (RPE) to gauge intensity rather than heart rate because it is much simpler and doesn't require any math or pulse counting. Ideally RPE should reach 16-19 during the higher-intensity intervals and 9-12 during the lower-intensity intervals.

The Borg RPE Scale
6 = Least Effort
7 = Very, Very Light
8
9 = Very Light
10
11 = Fairly Light
12
13 = Somewhat Hard
14
15 = Hard
16
17 = Very Hard
18
19 = Very, Very Hard
20 = Maximum Effort

Intensity, duration and recovery are interdependent. The harder you exercise the shorter you will be able to do it and the longer recovery period your body will require. So you may only be able to last **30 sec** at an RPE of 19 and require 3 minutes to recover, but you may be able to last two minutes at an RPE of 17 and only require one minute to recover.

The lower-intensity "recovery" period in between the higher-intensity intervals is called the base level. **The** base should be active recovery **so** no matter how out of breath you get during the high-intensity interval you should keep moving during recovery. Do not just stand still, sit or lie down. In fact, if you have to do any of these things then your interval was probably too intense (unless you are an athlete). Secondly, the optimal base level should be about an 11-13 (fairly light to somewhat hard) on the RPE scale. This will vary according to how hard the interval is. The harder the intervals are the easier the base level needs to be. Third, judge your base level intensity BEFORE you do any high-intensity intervals. Once you complete several intervals the base level is going to seem harder than it was at the beginning and that's normal. Lastly, it's okay to adjust your base level depending on how you are feeling. I often adjust my base level up or down depending on how I feel that day.

To increase intensity during the intervals you can go faster (sprints), harder (climbs), or a combination of the two (hills). The combinations of challenges (sprints, climbs and hills), intensities, interval periods, rest periods, modes (treadmill, elliptical cross-trainer, rower, bike, outdoor walking, swimming, etc.) and total workout time means you are totally in control of your routine. And for those who crave variety it means a virtually endless array of combinations so you really never even have to perform the same routine twice while still leading to amazing results.

HIIT for the Beginner

Here are some tips for those that are new to HIIT or are out of shape:

- Choose the cardio exercise that you feel the most comfortable with (treadmill, outdoor walking, stationary bike, elliptical, seated stepper, etc.)
- Experiment by exercising a little harder than usual until you feel like you are getting out of breath and then back off to your usual pace or even a little below it
- Note how you feel during the recovery period and when you have caught your breath then try it again
- Use longer intervals (2-3 minutes) and limit how hard you go during the higher-intensity intervals (RPE 16-17)
- The length of the recovery intervals should be longer than the higher-intensity intervals; shoot for a ratio of 1:2 or 1:3
- When you feel comfortable try one of our sample beginner routines

Beginner **HIIT** Workout # 1

Total time: 20min

Warm-Up (4:00) – Start easy and gradually increase exercise intensity so that you achieve an RPE of about 11-12 (this is your base level) by the end of the warm-up.

Stage 1 (9:00) 3 Hills

Hill #1: Increase speed and resistance/incline to an RPE of 15 for 1 minute. Return to base level for 2 minutes.

Repeat twice.

Stage 2 (4:00) 3 Sprints

Sprint #1: Increase speed to an RPE of 17 for 20 seconds. Return to base level for 60 seconds.

Repeat twice.

Cool-Down (3:00) – Decrease intensity to achieve an RPE of 9-10. Heart rate should return to within about 20-30 beats per minute of pre-exercise value.

Beginner HIIT Workout #2
Total time: 25min

Warm-Up (4:00) – Start easy and gradually increase exercise intensity so that you achieve an RPE of about 11-12 (this is your base level) by the end of the warm-up.

Stage 1 (12:00) 3 Climbs
Hill #1: Increase resistance/incline to an RPE of 15 for 2 minutes. Return to base level for 2 minutes.
Repeat twice.

Extra Recovery (1:00) – Stay at base level or adjust accordingly so that you are fully recovered for the next challenge.

Stage 2 (4:00) 4 Sprints
Sprint #1: Increase speed to an RPE of 17 for 20 seconds. Return to base level for 40 seconds.
Repeat three times.

Cool-Down (3:00) – Decrease intensity to achieve an RPE of 9-10. Heart rate should return to within about 20-30 beats per minute of pre-exercise value.

HIIT for the Experienced

Here are some tips for those that already perform cardio exercise on a regular basis and are in good shape:

- Try out one of the sample beginner programs to see how you respond
- Choose any mode of exercise that you are accustomed to but don't be afraid to experiment with new forms. For example, if you are having a difficult time challenging yourself while walking outside but don't want to jog or run (maybe due to joint issues) then try the elliptical trainer (allows greater increases in intensity while still being gentle on the joints)
- Play with the intervals and intensities to find out what works best for you and what you enjoy the most
- Mix up your HIIT routine so that you aren't always doing to same thing – keep it fresh and interesting, the possibilities are endless

Advanced HIIT Workout

Total Time: 32:30 min

Warm-Up (4:00) – Start easy and gradually increase exercise intensity so that you achieve an RPE of about 11-12 (this is your base level) by the end of the warm-up.

Stage 1 (7:30)
- Sprint for 2min at RPE 18 with 30sec recovery
- Hill for 2min at RPE 18 with 30 sec recovery
- Sprint for 2 min at RPE 18 with 30 sec recovery

Extra Recovery (1:00)

Stage 2 (5:00)

- Hill for 1 min at RPE 18 and 1 min at RPE 19-20 with 30 sec recovery
- Repeat

Extra Recovery (1:00)

Stage 3 (11:00)
- Hill for 3 min at RPE 17 with 60 sec recovery
- Max sprint for 30 sec with 60 sec recovery
- Repeat twice

Cool-Down (3:00) – Decrease intensity to achieve an RPE of 9-10. Heart rate should return to within about 20-30 beats per minute of pre-exercise value.

Never Grow Old!

Chapter 6: Holding your Own

We want to share with you just a few of the many inspirational stories we have witnessed over the years. We have seen clients with Parkinson's in their late 70s, who haven't gotten out of a chair unassisted in years. In fact, when we asked he and his wife how many years has it been, they both said "More years than I can even remember." That comment did get the client visibly teary and my tough macho trainer couldn't keep it together either. We have trained clients in their 80s into great physical shape so much so they still climb up on their own roof to clean out the gutters (just don't tell his wife). We have had clients like Sue (who is a model in this book) still showing six pack abs at age 55!   Clients who have won the first 5k they have ever run in their age group 45-55. We believe there are some principles you can take away from each of these stories even if they don't relate perfectly to your situation or fitness goals.

Howard: Start Early

I know when I first met Howard I was rather shocked to learn he was 92. Yes I have worked with people in their 60s, 70s, 80s and even 90s but I still have some presuppositions as to what 90 should look like. Howard didn't fit my stereotype. He wasn't frail. He didn't seem "old" at all, except that he moved slowly and deliberately, but even then it didn't look like he was struggling at all just that he didn't want to hurry. He was tremendously witty, and always had a joke (often dirty) to tell. Howard told me he had given up golfing a few years back so I asked him clarify at what age he had stopped. He said, "oh around age 88 or 89 I forget…..and not cause I forget things". In fact I don't think Howard forgot anything. With great detail he told me about all the sports legends from the 30s and 40s as clear as if it were yesterday.

Howard was also incredibly strong for someone in their nineties even though by his standards all of his strength had left him. You see he had spent so much time in his earlier years building up so much strength that what he had left in his 90s was actually beyond that of the average 60 year old. He told me how he used to throw 100 lb. bags of potatoes for hours loading trucks. I consider myself pretty strong, but throwing 100lbs around is a pretty physical task. He also played college sports and stayed physically active through his adulthood, again he didn't give up golf until his late 80s. He joked, "once I couldn't beat the young guys anymore it just wasn't as much fun". Of course I had to ask how young are the young guys? "Oh you know guys in their 60s and 70s". He had shot many a round under par in his younger days and so in his 70s and 80s was still beating players 20 years his junior.

So how does Howard's story relate to you? You see his body stayed strong and his mind stayed incredibly sharp until the very end of his life at the young age of 94. Sure he slowed down at the end, but he still walked on his own, went out for breakfast with the boys and out lived most of his contemporaries. He was able to do this because he had built a tremendous amount of physical reserve when he was younger so that even in his 90s he still had plenty of strength, stamina and energy to do everything he needed to do independently. The moral of this story is that if you are in your 50s or 60s now then make it a priority to get as functionally strong as you can so when you are 90 you will still be able to function independently and enjoy life to the very end just as Howard did.

Don: The kindergarten fitness goal

Probably the most unique yet simple fitness goal I have ever been asked to help achieve was that of tying ones shoes. Now I know you might be saying I already know how to tie my own shoes, what does this have to do with fitness? Well it really wasn't about the skill of tying shoes as it was about the physical ability to reach his feet again. Don came to me at age 72 and actually was in great physical shape. He exercised regularly and had for all his adult life. His main problem was that he had undergone 4 knee replacement surgeries (3 times on one knee and once on the other)! He was left with such stiffness and poor range of motion he couldn't get to his own feet to tie his shoes. I remember him saying "It is pretty embarrassing to make a nice 20 foot birdie putt and then feel like an old man asking for someone to pick my ball out of the hole for me." After about 4 weeks of range of motion exercises, some aggressive stretching and some balance training he came in one day and said, "Hey Dan check out my shoes!" He actually got me, I thought to myself this is odd…..guys my age don't ever say that….. pretty sure guys in their 70s don't care about new shoes……then it hit me, he isn't asking about the shoes. I looked down and saw nicely tied shoes instead of the special self scrunchy shoe laces he normally wore. I looked back up at Don and he was beaming. I think we both had tears in our eyes although neither of us will ever admit it. Sometimes the simplest things in life are also the sweetest.

Jessie: Inspirational at 80

Jessie is one of the models in this book and she has shown us time and time again that your 80s can be a beautiful and graceful decade. We far to often have negative thoughts about people in their 80s are sick or tired, or sick and tired, not pictures of energy, vitality, and certainly not doing 30 pushups or having even any aspirations to do that. Jessie has been an exerciser for decades and it shows. I think you can see several big smiles on her face in the photos. I routinely hear women that train with her (women in their 30s, 40s, 50s, and 60s) say I want be just like Jessie she rocks! I think what they are expressing is they are seeing that 80 year-olds can do what 30 year-olds can do if they really want that. I have a video of Jessie doing pushups, and that video was shot just a few months after she cracked some ribs! Pretty amazing most 80 year olds wouldn't be caught on film doing pushups with sore ribs. In fact, she begs forgiveness for only doing about a dozen and admittedly not her best pushups since she was a solid month out of practice. But again it displays her ability to bounce back from an injury because she had the physical strength available to her, plenty in her bank.

Lance: Train like the NFL

Lance is the only male model in our book, **demonstrating some of the bonus exercises,** and he continues to amaze and inspire me. He is an example of what level you can reach if you are willing and want to work hard. He has been training with us for about 2 years and he gives everything he has got. He routinely apologizes for getting tired and I have to remind him he is getting tired because I am training him so hard and people half his age would be tired. Recently, he commented to me about seeing a promotional video on the NFL combine and he remarked, "those NFL guys are doing many of the things we are doing in our training session? Am I doing the wrong program?" I smiled and said, "nope you have advanced to the highest level of functional movements so the same things they throw at NFL guys I am throwing at you, just be glad you don't have to get on the field and take the punishment their bodies take." Lance smirked and said "I think this training is about all the punishment this old body can take anymore......but seriously this is amazing to think I am doing some of the exercises those guys do."

Doug and Sidney: Adventure at any age!

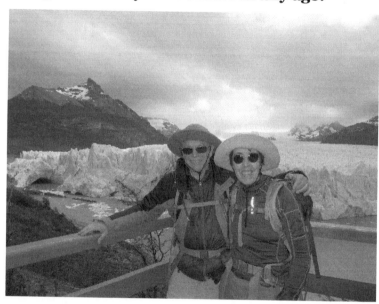

"Adventure travel is our passion. As seniors, personal training has made possible what heretofore only younger bodies dared to try. In fact, we had to get special permission to hike on this glacier here in Los Glaciares National Park in Patagonia since the "rules" don't allow anyone over 65 out on the ice. In spite of the steep pitches and dangerous footing, our personal training made the glacier hike, while challenging, very doable-- as well as a lifetime memory. We think personal training has added at least a decade to our adventure travel careers." Drs. Doug Sprenkle and Sidney Moon

From Dr. Summer

At age 55, I thought I was probably done with my mountain climbing career. I was somewhat of a casual climber having spent a bit of time in the Rockies and quite a bit of time in Alaska. My brother is a teacher in Kenai and so each summer we would get together for a hunting or fishing adventure, often spending a week hiking in the various ranges that make Alaska such a challenging destination. While crossing Alaska we would constantly be impressed by the image of Denali, the highest peak in North America, which seemed to challenge us each time we were in its vicinity. Eventually my brother decided he needed to face that challenge. He had had plenty of others - dealing with cancer as a young man and then the after effects of radiation which weakened his heart. He decided to put a climb together composed of cancer survivors with the intent of bringing awareness to the public and raising funds for children's cancer camps, one of which is here in Indiana. I decided I should go along, primarily to keep an eye on him, but also to push myself physically and mentally and support what I felt was a very worthwhile cause. I was just turning 40 and was in decent shape. By running and working out I thought I had myself adequately prepared for a 20,000 foot mountain and three long weeks of constant physical exertion. The climb was quite the adventure and my brother and I shared the exhilaration of standing together on the summit of one of the worlds most impressive mountains. I survived, but realized I had been fortunate. My training had been adequate but my preparation could have been better organized and more effective. I considered some other peaks, but really had been satisfied with my Denali effort and was not looking for another alpine adventure. My daughter however, thought otherwise. She is a public health worker in Uganda. A group had decided to climb Mt Kilimanjaro -again in a fund raising effort. This was an international group representing the UNICEF chapter based in the United Kingdom. The principle climbers were acquaintances of my daughter - friends she had met in Africa. Again, I felt an obligation to accompany a family member and keep them out of trouble while I shared the experience and supported a worthy cause. This time however, I felt I needed a bit more guidance in preparation for climbing another 20,000 foot peak in equatorial Africa. This is where Miracles Fitness and their staff came to my aid. I knew I needed a solid program geared toward endurance , strength, and agility. All of these factors had deteriorated in the 15 years since my Denali summit. I still felt I had the ability and the reserves to attempt this climb, but the last thing I wanted was to be unprepared. I was able to work with several of their training staff, all of whom were knowledgeable and thorough. I tried to work out three times a week at Miracles and then additional days on my own. But, I found I would not push myself enough on my own and required the 'encouragement' of my trainers to make the progress I needed. Mary Ehresman, in particular, seemed to take a special interest in my effort. Ultimately, I was able to keep up with the kids who made up the climbing party and shared another summit experience with my daughter on the top of Africa. Truly an experience I will never forget. And I don't think I could have done it without the months I spent training. I have in fact been so encouraged by my Kilimanjaro adventure, I am planning on climbing the Grand Teton in Wyoming this summer. I can hardly wait!

Thanks, Dan---- Tom Summer

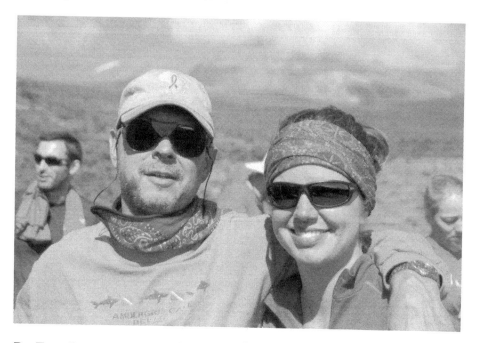

Dr. Tom Summer and his daughter Anna on their Mt Kilimanjaro adventure

A personal note from one client of ours from Linda:

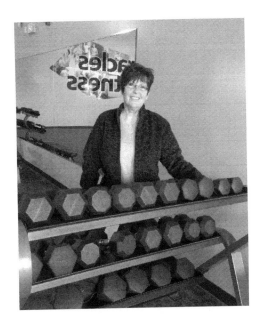

I retired in July of 2011. I am loving retirement , but I also knew that I needed to keep busy. Now it is time to do some things I wanted to, but never took the time.

Probably 75% of people make a resolution to get in shape by eating healthy and exercising more, in January 2012, I decided to do the same.

I joined Miracles Fitness and to my surprise I really loved it. I have dieted and exercised on and off my whole life (more off than on in the last 20 years). The trainers are absolutely awesome! I look forward to going and working out. These are words that I never thought would come out of my mouth! The workouts have encouraged me to watch my food intake as well.

One of the things I was really determined to do was, as that "65" came closer and closer, to not be on a punch of pills. It seems like you start on one and more just keep getting added. My blood pressure was borderline 148/78. I have been a member for just three short months and it is down to 120/80. I would be the last person in the world to say I can't miss my workout and now I am thrilled to say it and totally mean every word.

Now I arrange my schedule, for the most part, around my workout times. I have earned it and I want to be able to continue to be healthy.

As mothers and grandmothers, we have a right to be selfish and take this time for ourselves....everyone benefits! Miracles is a good name for the fitness center because I truly think it is a Miracle that it has become such a big part of my life!

--Linda Corbin--

Did you catch that second to last line, we have a right to be selfish....everyone benefits? Ponder this for a moment. How many people are impacted by your health or lack of it? How many generations may be impacted by you living well in your 70s, 80s and 90s? This point will be much of our focus for our final chapter. Aging well isn't just about you, it is about our society, our community and most definitely our family. Is it selfish to take care of your health and take time to exercise? Or is it selfish to not take care of yourself and let your body decline with age much faster or quicker than designed?

Aging successfully is much more about maintaining and holding on to as much physical function as possible than it is about turning back a magic clock. Aging successfully has significant impacts on those around us. My grandmother prays faithfully for her grandchildren (me) every day in her late 80s. I am pretty sure that when she is gone that won't be replaced. I will miss knowing that presence in my life. While her physical function is beginning to falter and I know she misses my late grandfather dearly, her presence still has an impact on those around her. My other grandmother is in her 90s and taught English as a 2nd language to Afghan refugee women crossing into Pakistan. She did this in her late 70s and early 80s until her church was bombed. I am sure someone somewhere said aren't you getting to old for this Winnie? I don't think that thought ever crossed her mind, it simply wasn't in her DNA.

Can You Imagine It?

For just a moment I want you to ponder this…..you have an age number in your head at which you expect your life will end.   It is in there whether you admit it or not so close your eyes and focus on what age you think you will be when you die.   Okay, got it?

Now add ten years to that number.

Now add 15 years to that number!

If you were to live 10 years or 15 years longer than you ever imagined how might your life need to change this year or this month or this week…or even today?

Chapter Take-Aways

People can live into their 90s and have a high quality of life.
You might live 10 years longer than you imagine.
Your fitness goals might have nothing to do with fitness, but everything to do with life, and life to its fullest.

Resource
www.functionalfitnesssolution.com

Conclusion

Dear Reader,

So now what are you to make of all of this? Can these functional exercises not only add years to my life, but enhance the quality of those years? What if I live to be 10 years older than I can even imagine? These are questions we really want you to think deeply about. We believe the research is very clear that the aging process can be positively impacted by the right kinds of exercise. The trajectory you are on for your functional ability in your 70s, 80s and 90s is directly related to the actions you are taking right now with respect to physical training to maintain your body.

It is tempting to think that we have nothing left to accomplish in the last 20 years of our life and that our "best" or more productive years will be behind us. If that is so then why bother to put in all of this effort with an exercise program now? We want to share an inspiring story about a man you have probably all heard about who made his biggest accomplishments in his mid to late 70's. He was in prison for 27 years from the age of 45 (1962) to the age of 72 (1990). During those years he experienced horrible conditions, inadequate food, and most likely abusive treatment. But despite all of that he maintained a regular regime of pushups, sit-ups and running in place. There was a 3 year period where he was in a shared cell large enough to run small laps much to the annoyance of his fellow cell-mates. After being released from prison (at the age of 72) he rejoined the political movement he had started over 25 years earlier. Three years later Nelson Mandela was elected president of South Africa and was eventually awarded the Nobel Peace Prize.

It is safe to conclude that his 27 year fitness regimen significantly contributed to his significance and success upon release. If Nelson Mandela had emerged from prison a frail, weak, broken "old" man he certainly would not have been able to become the inspirational leader for his country and the rest of the world that he is fondly remembered for. We could say that the most productive years of his life were taken from him or we could say that age is just a number...one that shouldn't hold us back from being the best that we can be.

What do you have yet to accomplish? A major achievement in your field? Amazing adventures? Dancing with your granddaughter at her wedding? Whatever your endeavor we know you have a significant purpose or calling for every single one of your remaining years. We hope this program helps you to live those years with more gusto, energy, enthusiasm, and joy than you ever thought possible.

Sincerely,

Dan and Cody

About The Authors

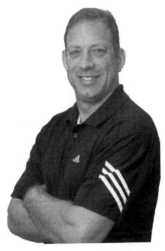

Cody Sipe, PhD

Cody is an award-winning, 20 year veteran of the fitness industry, a professor of Physical Therapy, exercise specialist and recognized authority on exercise for mature adults. He earned his Master's Degree in Exercise Science from Virginia Teach and his PhD in Exercise Science from Purdue University. He is co-owner of Miracles Fitness and has helped thousands of older adults improve their health and well-being through the numerous exercise programs and facilities which he has been a part of. Cody co-founded the Functional Aging Institute to offer programs for Fitness Professionals around the world who are interested in training mature clients. For his innovative work he was awarded the International Program Director of the Year Award in 2005 from the IDEA Health and Fitness Association (one of the largest membership organizations for fitness professionals in the world). Cody is the proud father of 7 children (Cassie, Carter, Caden, Colson, Callie, Cortlyn and Collins) and husband of 1 wife (Jenny). He enjoys coaching sports teams for his children, hiking, exercising, travelling, and public speaking. He is passionate about ethnic, weird, unusual or exotic foods and looks for every excuse to try something new (thank you Anthony Bourdain and Andrew Zimmern). His love of great coffee is well-known to his family and friends and one of his favorite gifts to receive will always be a Starbucks gift card.

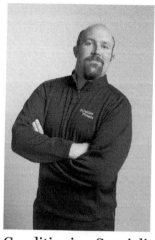

Dan Ritchie, PhD

Dan is the co-owner of Miracles Fitness in West Lafayette and Lafayette Indiana. He was a Lynn Fellow at Purdue University completing his PhD in Health and Kinesiology with a minor in Gerontology. He has served on several boards including the Midwest American College of Sports Medicine Board of Directors and the American College of Sports Medicine Student Affairs Committee. He is a Certified Strength and Conditioning Specialist, from NSCA, and a Health Fitness Specialist from ACSM, as well as a Master Trainer for Enhance Fitness, a widely recognized evidenced based exercise program. In 2013 Dan co-founded the Functional Aging Institute a company committed to educating Fitness Professionals around the world.

Dan is originally from the Chicago area and has been married to his wife Jenifer for almost 20 years. They have 5 children (Luke, Ethan, Caleb, Elena, and Ryan). Dan has always enjoyed playing just about every sport. He and his family love to visit Colorado regularly and hike in the mountains, exploring for moose and bear.

Resources

We encourage you to visit our blog at www.functionalfitnesssolution.com/blog for new exercise routines, videos, tips, articles, interviews and discussions of concepts and best practices related to healthy aging and fitness.

For more exercise programs please visit our website: www.functionalfitnesssolution.com

For fitness professionals seeking more education please visit our website: www.functionalaginginstitute.com

We would love to hear from you. Please send us your comments, feedback and questions concerning the Never Grow Old Exercise Program or any related topic.

How to Contact Us:

By email:

DrCodySipe@Gmail.com
DanMRitchie@Gmail.com

Functional Fitness Solution
257 Sagamore Pkwy West
West Lafayette, IN 47906

If you are interested in Affiliate and commissions opportunities to promote our products please email us directly.

Made in the USA
Lexington, KY
07 July 2014